MISS GLORIA

Allie Cormier

MISS GLORIA

A SURVIVOR
OF TERRORISM

ELLEN BOMER

WITH MARY MCNEIL

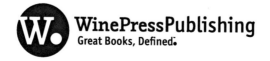

WinePressPublishing
Great Books, Defined.

WinePress Publishing (PO Box 428, Enumclaw, WA 98022) functions only as book publisher. As such, the ultimate design, content, editorial accuracy, and views expressed or implied in this work are those of the author.

All Scripture quotations, unless otherwise indicated, are taken from the *New King James Version*®. Copyright © 1982 by Thomas Nelson, Inc. Used by permission. All rights reserved.

ISBN 13: 978-1-4141-1366-1
ISBN 10: 1-4141-1366-8
Library of Congress Catalog Card Number: 2008910933

June,

To my husband, Don,
my sons, John and Michael,
and the peace that comes from knowing
the presence of God

Live, Love, Laugh

Ellen Boman   5-16-11

CONTENTS

Acknowledgments. ix

Prologue xi

Foreword. xiii

1. The Phone Call 1
2. From the Mountain. 9
3. To the Valley 15
4. Aftershocks 23
5. Survivor. 27
6. Boot Camp for the Blind 57
7. ABC Nightline and LCB Graduation. 67
8. Orange Juice Never Looked Better 85
9. The Trial 93
10. From the Ashes 107
11. When Positive is Negative. 115

12. A New Outlook 121
13. In Their Own Words 127
14. ". . . But God Meant It for Good . . ." 139

Resources 141

Endnotes 145

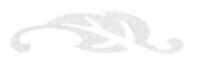

ACKNOWLEDGMENTS

M Y HEARTFELT THANKS and appreciation go out to:

My husband, Don, for his support throughout this ordeal and for his diligence in chronologically detailing the events, which made the writing of this book so much easier.

Our dear friends Jan Kauffman and Sharon Carter for professionally editing with inclusion of my spiritual feelings. Their creativity, talent and insight are remarkable.

My brother, George Karas, for his efforts in researching and preparing a proposal for this book.

My many friends and co-workers in the Department of Commerce who did everything in their power to see that my care was the best available; those who sent hundreds of e-mails, cards, letters, flowers; and those who called and visited me. I will never forget you.

All medical and support personnel at Landstuhl Army Medical Center and Walter Reed Army Medical Center for their professionalism and compassionate care for me and the other survivors. Their task of caring for us physically, mentally, emotionally, and spiritually was indeed daunting. I have nothing but praise for all who tended to me during that time, from the commanders down to the privates. These were truly MY heroes!

The Military Airlift Command (MAC). Especially the crews that flew me and my comrades from Nairobi to Germany and on to the U.S.

All organ donors who gave me a chance at regaining my sight and to others, life itself.

Rhonda Hayman for transcribing my dictation in the course of writing this book.

And last, but not least, my dear friend and running buddy Nancy Cooper who passed from this mortal life in early 2010. We shopped, traveled, laughed, and cried together so often. I miss you, girl, but I know I'll see you again in heaven.

PROLOGUE

MOSES, THE KENYAN driver, and I stood in our office on the ground floor at the rear of the embassy building.

Pop, pop!

Moses jumped onto the air conditioner unit to get a better look.

Then blackness . . .

As I regained consciousness, I thought, *A bomb!*

Then my mind turned to my physical condition. I tried to turn over or sit up, but couldn't. I was lying flat on my back, my torso pinned securely to the floor, only my legs, arms, and head free to move. I imagined I knew what an overturned sea turtle must feel like.

Worse than feeling like a beached amphibian, I realized I couldn't see. *Please God, don't let me be blind!* I started bargaining with God. *Let me have one eye; You can have the other; just let me have one.*

I removed something from my mouth and heard water trickling. *Oh, please, God, don't let me drown.*

Fear and anxiety rose inside me, but I knew I had to remain calm. *Don't panic; don't panic. God, give me strength; God, give me strength!*

Just then I heard movement. Waving my right arm, I called out, "I'm over here! Please, I'm over here!"

In 1998, I was one of the Americans who survived the explosion of the Nairobi U.S. Embassy terrorist bombing linked to the Arab-Afghan al-Qaeda run by Saudi financier, Osama bin Laden: the elusive terrorist leader who later destroyed New York City's Twin Towers in 2001.

In alarming news heard 'round the world, the Associated Press reported that two U.S. embassies were successfully targeted in Africa: one in Nairobi, Kenya, and the other in Dar es Salaam, Tanzania. Two hundred twenty-four were killed and over 5,000 injured, the majority in the Nairobi attack. As an American employee, I nearly died when the embassy walls caved in on me, pinning me down in a semi-conscious state for over five hours, until I was finally rescued. Under covert security protection, my code name became "Miss Gloria." This begins as my story, and ultimately becomes the story of the many who played a role in saving my life on the long road to recovery.

FOREWORD

HOW MANY OF you have wished for a second chance? After the bombing I knew I was in the presence of God, and I knew I was not going to die. He said, *"Ellen, go back and let them heal you."* The peace and the awe and the grandeur around me . . . mere words can't describe it. After all the pain, the suffering, the surgeries, the physical therapy, we went back to Alabama, and in 2001 my granddaughter, Alexandra Cormier, was born.

Throughout the aftermath of the bombing, I kept thinking, *I'm useless. I'm blind. There is nothing I can do, Lord. What is it You want me to do? There is nothing I can do. I love You, but surely there is a purpose. What do You want me to do?* Well, on August twenty-six, my doorbell rang. A woman from social services stood there with my two-week-old granddaughter, and asked if I would take her. She put her in my arms and I cradled this baby to my breast. I was terrified. I couldn't even see her. Where am I going to put this child? How am I going to feed her? How am I going to bathe her? How am I going to take care of her?

But then joy took over! *Okay, I can do this. I can do this!*

So I took the baby in and she became mine. I changed her diapers. I prepared her formula by myself. I fumbled; I bumbled; but with the help of God, I did it.

Allie was an excellent baby. She never cried. When I bathed her for the first time, I took her into the bathroom and put her into a sink that had a console on it. I thought, *Okay, if I drop her she can't go far. It's only five inches deep.* I held her by one hand and put her little "heinie" in it, washing her up: soap-soap-soap, lotion, and powder—then lifted her into my arms and breathed, "Whew, I did it. I did it. She's okay."

So on we went. She started crawling. Well, if any of you have been around toddlers, you know they are pretty active, and I'm still this bumbling blind person. My solution was bells on her shoes. When she progressed to her knees, I hovered on top of her like this hulking bear on all fours. As she moved, I moved. We went all over that house. Back and forth; back and forth for hours and hours until she got too fast for me. Then I couldn't keep up with her, but I had bells to follow. When it came time for her to talk and walk, Allie would grab Suzie's tail (Suzie is our French Poodle) and Suzie would haul her around the house. It was so cute. I could hear her while Allie laughed.

When it came time to feed her something besides a bottle, well, you know that is a chore, even if you can see. So I put the child in the high chair, and I thought, *Okay, this is real easy.* But I couldn't find her. I couldn't find her in the high chair! When at last I found her, I reached for the spoon, but then I couldn't find the spoon. I knew this wasn't going to work. My solution was to sit down on the barstool with Allie's back to my chest. I put a big old-fashioned white diaper around her like a barber shop chair. I held her chin in my hand and started shoveling. Before long her little mouth would be wide open looking for that spoon. And now I can surely say that she is healthy, alive, and well. We both did fine throughout it all!

Allie was baptized when she was eleven months old. When she was two years old in 2004, we moved to Wimberley, Texas. As she turned three, I knew she had to have some interaction with other children. So I found St. Stephen's Episcopal School, which had a daycare school two or three days a week for little ones. So I brought Allie to daycare twice a week.

She loved it! She was like a little bloom that they were watering with kindness, love, discipline, and Christ. She was blooming. Don and I thought, *Well, this is really neat. Let's check out this church.*

I was a Catholic for fifty-four years, and Catholics did not go to other churches. Don was Presbyterian. He now agreed to go with me to this one, because I was blind and I could not go by myself.

This is how we came to be part of St. Stephen's Episcopal Church. Allie would go to the nursery, while Don and I went to the service. That was wonderful, and because Allie was baptized, I coached her about communion. I told her how important it was to receive the Eucharist inviting Christ within you. So then we started bringing Allie from the nursery for communion. Before communion Father Ted Knies, the officiating priest, called all the little children up to him. Allie toddled up with the others, and they all sat on the floor while he talked with them. It put me in mind of Christ when He said, "Bring the children unto me." I thought, *This IS a man of God; we need to be here.* Then we took communion.

Eucharist is extremely important to me. It's the one time I have sight. I kneel at the altar, and receive our Lord. And He is with me. When I received the Eucharist for the first time at St. Stephen's, it was like, *Oh, my God, You're with me again. I'm here and You're here with me.* As I returned to my seat, knelt down, and started praying, I was filled with the notion: *Stay here, Ellen, and let them heal you!* After that, all my prayers and all my vapor went up to the heavens, and the water came down and showered me with His love and blessings.

CHAPTER 1

THE PHONE CALL

LIFE WAS GOOD. My husband, Don, and I were settled in our home in Huntsville, Alabama, after having spent several years living and working in Germany in the late seventies.

We first met at social gatherings held in apartment complexes. Don came to one of these single parties with a date and I was the greeter. I noticed that he was tall, with blue eyes, and had a beautiful voice. A couple of weeks later I went to another function and saw him come in with a different woman. It appeared they were together. Well, Don kept asking me to dance and if I wanted something to drink. I thought to myself, *That's really tacky!* So finally I asked, "What about the woman you brought?" to which he replied, "We only walked in at the same time." She wasn't his date! I felt a lot better. It was very nice to dance with someone who was taller than I.

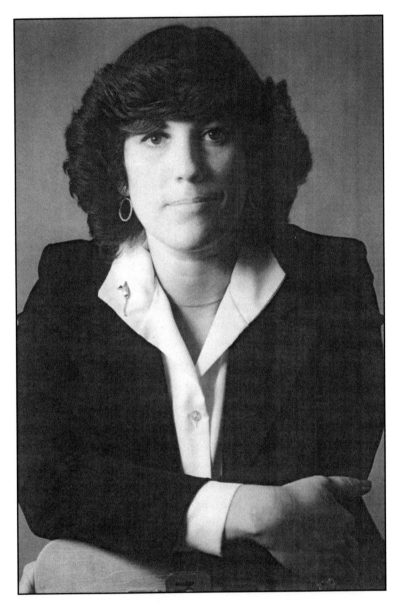

Ellen Bomer – 1977

We were happily married for thirteen years, with two teenage boys getting along well (finally!), and I had graduated from college with a degree in Business Administration and Economics in 1984.

One major concern remained, however. My son, John, had struggled throughout his childhood and teenage years with emotional and physical problems, as well as learning disabilities. Even though I, as his mother, saw so much potential in him, he didn't always see it in himself. He had graduated from high school, but couldn't seem to find his niche. For several months I prayed regularly for him, "Lord, please help John to find his place." At this time, I felt very close to God. A co-worker invited me to a Wednesday night prayer service. The entire service consisted of singing. I did this for six months religiously for an hour each week. As we sang, I prayed with my heart to God. Tears would stream down my face. I know my prayers were answered.

At Christmastime in 1986, our typical holiday routine was disrupted. We're a social family, and we normally went to several parties and hosted a few of our own. This year, however, we were all sick—stay in pajamas all day, lie on the couch, sip hot tea sick. Because of that, we were forced to stay home and simply spend time with each other. We didn't realize at the time what a precious gift that sickness was!

Just after the New Year, I made a rare trip north to visit distant relatives in hopes of renewing our relationship. The

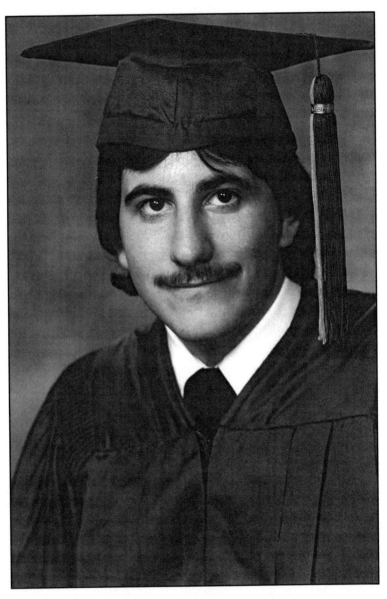

Our son John at graduation (1986)

night before I left, John said to me, "Mom, wake me up and kiss me good-bye before you go tomorrow."

"I'm leaving so early," I replied. "You don't really want me to wake you, do you?"

"Yes. Promise?"

So, as promised, the following morning before dawn I woke my son, hugged him, and told him I loved him.

That was the last time I saw my son alive.

While I was visiting my aunts and cousins, John went to Tennessee to help a friend move.

The evening after I returned home, we got a call from John.

"Hey, Mom, just wanted to let you know I'll be home later tonight."

"I can't wait to see you," I said.

That day it had snowed heavily in both Tennessee and northern Alabama—an unusual weather pattern for the South. I told John to be careful driving on slippery roads as we said good-bye.

Around midnight the phone rang.

The caller identified himself as a Tennessee state trooper, and said, "We need you to drive up here. Your son's been in a car accident."

"Is he okay?"

"Well, he's badly injured, and you need to come."

Both Don and I had been sleeping soundly before the call came, so it took a few moments for the trooper's words to sink in. Once they did, however, we wasted no time in getting dressed and out the door.

In the hospital, they ushered us into a room where a chaplain sat waiting. As soon as I saw the minister, I thought, *My son is dead.* I don't know how, but I knew John was dead. My prayer that John would find his niche had been answered, but that place was not on earth. God had taken him, and confirmation would come later.

The chaplain confirmed my worst fear, and went on to relay the circumstances. En route home, John's car suffered a flat tire, and he had pulled off the highway to change it. He turned on his emergency flashers, set out a reflective triangle, and jacked up the car. The semi-truck driver said later that he saw John and his car from a distance away, but nonetheless, heard a thump and realized he'd hit him. John was killed instantly.

My mind didn't want to process this information. *I had just spoken with my son a few hours ago. How could he be dead?*

My faith in God is strong, but as we drove back home that night, I couldn't help but think God had answered my prayer in a cruel and spiteful way. I said to Him, "I asked You to help John find his place. Was there no place for him on earth? Did You have to take him away? Did I pray my son *dead*?" My anguish was the expression of my grief at losing him, but the central question in my heart was, *Where is my son? God, is he in heaven with You?*

For months afterward, every morning when I got in my car to go to work, I would cry. I wept from the depths of my soul for thirty minutes—all the way to the office. Then I'd dry my tears, work all day, and get back into my car to go home. As soon as I turned the key, I'd begin crying again, and I didn't stop until I pulled into our driveway.

The idea that I had "prayed my son dead" continued to torment me, until I finally sought the counsel of our priest. He assured me that my prayers were not responsible for John's death. He said, "Ellen, it doesn't work that way. And just think; the first person who held your son after he died was Christ. Our Lord cradled him in his arms. And John is waiting in heaven now for you."

Eleven years later, the words of the priest were confirmed.

CHAPTER 2

FROM THE
MOUNTAIN

NO MATTER HOW excruciating pain can be, life really does go on. And while I'm not sure if time actually heals anything, let alone our deepest wounds, its passage hopefully softens the sharp edges of our losses.

In 1990, Don accepted an exciting job opportunity, and we moved to Riyadh, Saudi Arabia, where we lived during Desert Shield and Desert Storm.

After a few months in our new environment, we were rudely awakened, in January 1991, by the blasts of scud missiles shaking our villa. According to later reports, the missiles had been successfully engaged by Patriot batteries, but it was a frightening experience, nonetheless. For the next several months, I had to carry a gas mask to and from work every day. And at night we huddled in the strongest part of our home when wailing sirens signaled another attack.

Don and I transferred to Jeddah, on the Red Sea, in 1993, where I took a position with the U.S. Department of Commerce and worked in the Commercial Office attached to the U.S. Consulate General in Jeddah. When Don wasn't totally immersed in computers outside of his job, we had a very active social life. We went out to dinner with other couples at least twice a week. We played bridge once a week. And even the U.S. Consulate in Jeddah had a weekly "Happy Hour."

Following the 1995 car bomb in Riyadh, which killed five Americans, and then the 1996 attack on the Khobar Towers in Dhahran, security personnel from Washington, D.C., arrived in Jeddah to beef up security measures at the consulate, and prepare employees and staff in case of a terrorist attack.

For a full week, we went through simulated terrorist attacks, drilling, responding, and learning procedures. Part of the time, I had to be "injured," and in a weird foreshadowing, my assigned injury was that I had glass in my eyes.

Once our "war games" wrapped up, we went back to business as usual, and all was calm in Jeddah.

Although we felt reasonably safe in our offices on the consulate grounds, the location was less than ideal. First, we were occupying rented mobile-home-type buildings, which weren't particularly comfortable or professional in appearance. Second, our location in the city didn't allow us to operate at peak effectiveness.

The Commercial Office exists to promote American business in foreign countries. We set up trade agreements between the USA and other countries and make travel arrangements for local businesspeople who need to travel to the United States to conduct business with U.S. corporations. In other words, the Commercial Office functions as a combination chamber of commerce plus travel agency. Therefore, it's essential that we have hands-on contact with local businesses.

To accommodate that need, our office relocated to a commercial center about five miles from the consulate in March 1998. I was very involved with the move, locating potential new properties, procuring new office furniture, equipment, and even a security system. Responsibilities included managing the building, inventory, and personnel. And because my efforts were successful, I was also asked by our Washington office if I would be willing to go to Nairobi, Kenya, and duplicate the process.

I was flattered and thrilled. It seemed too good to be true. I received all the necessary immunizations and began taking anti-malaria medication.

I had always wanted to go to Africa, but Don did not share my desire. So I made the journey on my own, and was greeted at the Nairobi airport on July 6, 1998, by my supervisor, Danny DeVito. He checked me into the Hilton Hotel, saying he would meet me in the lobby in the morning and take me to the American Embassy to meet my coworkers.

I didn't sleep well that night—or any night I stayed at the Hilton. The hotel is located downtown, right next to a major street. Traffic noise continued all night long, security seemed lax, and I felt very exposed and vulnerable.

After a few days at the embassy, I attended a security briefing. The facilitator stressed repeatedly that the only major issue the embassy faced was crime, stealing mostly. Many people in Nairobi are unemployed and poor, so we were told to never wear jewelry or travel with our car windows down.

Having experienced the terrorist attack simulation in Jeddah, I was quite skeptical of the rosy picture the speaker painted. The embassy in Nairobi had no "standoff" (sometimes called standoff distance or standoff zone), meaning, the closest distance a threat can come to a building. Anyone could walk or drive right up to the door. Being the "new kid," however, I kept my thoughts to myself.

I was extremely fortunate to arrive in Nairobi when I did. The Community Liaison Office had planned a women's weekend getaway to Lamu, an island off the coast of Kenya, accessible only by airplane and boat.

What an adventure! Twelve of us shared six bungalows. Our beds were swathed in mosquito netting, just like in the movies, and I felt as though Katharine Hepburn or Humphrey Bogart might appear at any moment.

Once we were all settled in our bungalows, we set off to explore the island. There are no vehicles on Lamu, so our adventure was purely foot-powered. We walked the seemingly endless beaches, while white, fluffy clouds strolled lazily across a brilliant blue sky, the sun warming our backs as we trudged along the pale white sand dunes. On the shoreline, the waves licked at our heels. Sand crabs scurried away, as sand dollars dug deeper into the wet sand of receding waves. Seeing the clear, sparkling waters of the Indian Ocean filled me with peace, and I felt so blessed to be in that place at that time.

Toward late afternoon we made our way back to the hotel and cleaned up. By then the sun had set, so the other women and I relaxed on the veranda and admired the star constellations while awaiting the arrival of our meals.

The hotel chef specialized in creating fresh seafood dishes, so my roommate and I shared a seafood feast. We had a huge lobster, plump meaty scallops, and crabs as large as salad plates. We hardly made a dent in the platter and then passed it around for all to share. After dinner we moved back to the veranda to watch a lunar eclipse. The whole day—and the rest of the weekend—was magical. I was experiencing my African fantasy come true.

On Sunday, we returned to Nairobi. As the plane passed Mount Kilimanjaro, I was awestruck by the peak's magnificent snow-capped summit rising above the clouds. I did not realize then, how soon I would descend from this mountaintop experience, into the valley of the shadow of death.

Monday morning, the embassy buzzed with anticipation for the upcoming visit of Secretary of the Treasury Robert Rubin. I was in charge of setting up security, and made sure the secretary would be accommodated in the Serena Hotel, which has a great standoff distance and is far more secure than the Hilton. Everyone pitched in to make his experience positive and profitable, our common goal forging an efficient and well-run team. I was proud to be a part of this group, if only for a short period.

After the secretary left, Danny and I petitioned to be moved from the Hilton to the Serena. We were given junior suites, and we both rested easier in these more comfortable and secure surroundings.

Weekends in Nairobi were filled with sightseeing trips, and every Tuesday night the girls who had gone to Lamu shared pasta together. My coworkers and I visited the home of Joy Adamson—of *Born Free* fame—now an education center and wildlife observation area. We also toured the house where *Out of Africa* was filmed. After that trip, I hosted a girls' pasta night, where we all watched the movie, crying and laughing together. That evening holds a special place in my heart, because less than forty-eight hours later, two of these precious women died, victims of the anger and hatred of terrorists.

Of course, none of us could have anticipated the darkness that lay ahead as we immersed ourselves in gathering as many sights and experiences as our senses could hold.

Before long a location was chosen for the new commercial office. Negotiations were underway with the property owner and the contracting officer at the envoy. The details had been pretty well taken care of, and I had nearly met all of my goals.

I was scheduled to depart Nairobi on August 6 and return to Jeddah. However, my supervisor asked me to delay my departure for two weeks and assist the commercial staff in arranging conferences for the upcoming visit of Secretary of Commerce William Daley, who was bringing a delegation of American businessmen seeking business partners in Kenya.

The request seemed reasonable, and I was glad to use my experience and talents to make the secretary's visit more enjoyable and profitable.

So I went into the American Embassy on August 7, 1998, with a smile on my face and a cheerful heart, never dreaming that consenting to delay my departure would change my life forever.

CHAPTER 3

TO THE VALLEY

I ARRIVED AT the embassy thinking about my weekend plans to visit one of the nearby game parks. I was looking forward to one last opportunity to observe Africa's exotic and fascinating wildlife before I headed back to Jeddah.

Moses, my Kenyan driver, greeted me as I entered our office, located on the ground floor at the rear of the building. Actually, the floor of our office was about five feet below ground level and our transom-like windows were about six and a half feet from the floor. Moses was a slightly built Christian man who was very caring. He was the sole provider for his family, which included his wife and baby, as well as his mother and father. His baby was about six or seven months old at this time. A good and gentle person, he always wore a smile on his face.

My friend Susan Wiley, who worked in the Community Liaison Office, stopped in to ask if she could use the copier. Hers was broken and she had to prepare information packets for the delegation Secretary Daley was bringing. While the machine spit out pages, we chatted.

"Do you really think we're safe in this embassy?" Susan asked me.

"No, I don't think so," I replied. "Security keeps telling us our only threat is crime, but this embassy is just not constructed with safety in mind. After what I learned during my security training in Saudi Arabia, I'd have to say this is a pretty soft target. If I were a terrorist, this is the place I'd bomb."

"Well, let's hope the terrorists don't know what you know." Susan straightened her copies and turned to leave. "I'll be back about noon to pick you up, okay?" She and I had planned to take the afternoon off to shop.

"Sounds good. See you then."

Susan closed the door and left.

A few minutes later, I asked Moses about his new baby, but before he could answer, we heard *pop! pop!* Moses jumped up onto the air conditioner unit to get a better look.

Then blackness . . .

As I drifted in the darkness, I dreamt about younger days when I attended St. Mary's Catholic boarding school in Mobile, Alabama, in the 1960s – from eighth through eleventh grades. The school was right across the street from the Cathedral of the Immaculate Conception. We had a band and marched in the Mardi Gras parades in Mobile each year.

When I would feel lonely, or wanted to talk to some kind of parental figure, no one was available. So I often prayed to St. Joseph, who was a father figure for me. I was very devoted to Catholicism and went to mass every day. This was my family. The bishop knew us all by name.

My mother and father divorced when I was ten years old, and I did not hear from my father again until I was nineteen. So there was no male role model in my life. Since I had no immediate family in Mobile, I stayed at the school with many other students. On holidays most of the students went home, but I only left the school occasionally. Out of the twelve in my dorm there might only be four left, including me. My mother was in another state. I would read and go to the chapel and say the rosaries. I said a lot of rosaries. The chapel was always open, priests and nuns coming and going between prayers.

As a child I was very quiet. I always felt like I was on the outside looking in. I wasn't unhappy, but I wasn't a gregarious joiner. My feelings were hurt easily and I felt pretty vulnerable most of the time. I prayed a lot. That was the type of environment I was in— surrounded by praying nuns.

In the evening, we had study period from 7:00 P.M. to 8:00 P.M.; then we could watch TV for about a half hour, and "lights out" was 9:00 P.M. sharp. We would kneel on wooden floors by our beds to pray, then get into bed and say the rosary. The other girls in the boarding school were my family. On a couple of rare occasions, I got to visit the home of one of the other girls. Obtaining permission from my mother to leave the school premises was very difficult.

I often prayed to St. Joseph and to God the Father. God has never been vengeful in my mind. And they were real to me.

As I regained consciousness, I thought, *A bomb!*

Then my mind turned to my physical condition. I tried to turn over or sit up but couldn't. I was lying flat on my back, my torso pinned securely to the floor, with only my legs, arms, and head free to move. I imagined I knew what an overturned sea turtle must feel like.

Worse than feeling like a beached amphibian, I now realized I couldn't see. *Please, God, don't let me be blind!* I started bargaining with God. *Let me have one eye. You can have the other; please let me have just one.*

I removed something from my mouth and heard water trickling. *Oh, please, God, don't let me drown.*

Fear and anxiety rose inside me, but I knew I had to remain calm. *Don't panic; don't panic. God, give me strength; God, give me strength!*

I must have drifted in and out of consciousness, because even though I was unaware of it at the time, I learned later that I was pinned down for several hours before I was found.

Finally I heard rustling noises. Waving my right arm, I called out, "I'm over here! Please, I'm over here."

I began to feel movement around me and knew I was getting help. Strangely, I don't remember hearing voices, and to this day, am not certain who rescued me.

Someone pulled my left arm and I screamed in pain. I felt hands lifting me out of the debris and placing me on a stretcher. I could feel my rescuers struggling with my weight. I apologized, "I'm sorry I'm so heavy. I'm sorry I'm so heavy."

I still could not see, and continued pleading with God to please let me have at least one eye. *I could get by with one eye*, I told Him.

The men placed my stretcher in the back of a truck and secured it. As we sped along the streets of Nairobi, it seemed as though we hit every pothole. The frantic movement of the truck brought me to a new awareness of what it means to live in the moment; time stood still and all I knew was a world of complete pain. It washed over me and wouldn't go away. Every pothole brought it to burning life.

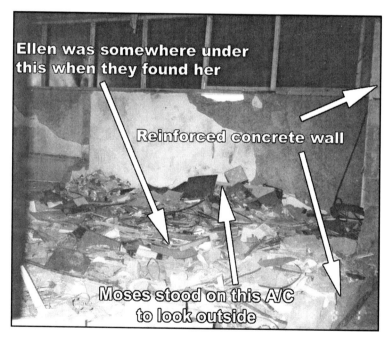

Office where Ellen was injured and Moses was killed[5]

I was taken to the Nairobi Medical Clinic, where I heard someone say, "This is an American from the embassy." Another responded, "Take her to Nairobi Hospital," and

I was painfully moved via another vehicle across town once again.

When we arrived at the hospital, I heard voices that I recognized. I remember thinking, *Thank God I'll be okay.* The embassy nurse told me that there had been a truck bomb attack on the embassy. Many people had been hurt, but the hospital staff would take care of me.

A short time later, Gretchen McCoy, the embassy doctor, came by to see me, then Ambassador Bushnell and my friend Susan. Susan's calm and soothing voice reassured me and made me feel safer and more confident. I remember telling Susan the combination to the safe in my hotel room and asking her to call Don and tell him where I was.

Susan left, and a stranger, newly assigned to the Nairobi embassy, came and held my hand. She became, on that significant occasion, the one who helped hold my fear at bay. I was so afraid; I did not believe I'd be able to handle the fear on my own if she left. I begged her again and again, "Please, don't leave me, please." This angel of mercy stayed with me as long as she could with her hand in mine, keeping me from being swept away by terror and panic. I never did find out her name, but to this day, I'm grateful for her kind and calming presence.

As I was moved into another room, the next thing that happened to me was everything going from grey to black . . . much darker than before, and totally silent. Lying there, I remember thinking to myself, *Oh God, if this is what it's like to die, I can do this. I can do this.* Such peace came over me that I had no pain. I had no fear. It was just wonderful peace.

Then the darkness started to brighten. Light began penetrating this darkness. It went from black to grey, and from grey it became brighter, brighter, and brighter until it became as intense as a white spotlight. I could see. And as I looked around, I saw people walking around me dressed alike. Different colors, but all the same. And they had regular American haircuts. These were people I knew! People I was comfortable around. And I remember saying, "Turn your head so I can see your face. I know you! Turn your head!" But nobody would turn. They were just walking around talking to each other; strolling by like it was an afternoon walk in the park.

I remember looking over my left shoulder to my left, and as I looked, there stood my deceased son, John. He was about four feet off the ground, floating there with his arms outstretched toward me like Christ to His followers. And he had that quirky smile on his face. It was just so peaceful and so loving. I knew it was him and I knew he was an angel in heaven because he was clean shaven. The mustache that he always wore had been previously shaved off at the funeral home.

I thought to myself, *Oh, John, you're here; you're here.* I reached out with my left arm, which was in a sling. I could actually see the sling around it, as I extended this arm off the side of the gurney I was lying on. I stretched it out almost totally horizontal like a "T," as John continued smiling with his arms reaching toward me. Then, as I was about to touch him . . . I was maybe an inch away . . . everything stopped.

I was sucked back, seeing strange shapes fly by me as if I were going through a worm hole in a sci-fi movie. I remember feeling instant loss . . . *Oh, no . . . please, I want to stay . . . I want to stay! This is so wonderful. I want to stay with you.* And I was told, "No, Ellen, it's not your time. You have to go back and let them heal you." And that's what I did.

21

Darkness enveloped me again, but I also immediately knew—beyond any shadow of doubt—that John was with God, and it wasn't my time to go. I also knew I was to be patient and let the medical staff take care of me. I remember accepting that but, never one to give up, I asked God again, *"Please let me have at least one eye; I can live with that."*

CHAPTER 4

AFTERSHOCKS

A T THE TIME, of course, I had no idea of the extent of my injuries. I learned later that I had suffered third-degree burns to my face, and hundreds of small shrapnel wounds to my head, face, shoulders, arms, hands, and legs—all on the front of the body. I also had a large, though not deep, cut on each foot. My eyes suffered the most damage, however. My right eye had been penetrated three times, and my left eye was perforated. The piece of glass, stone, or wood went completely through and is still embedded in my eye socket to this day.

The doctors in Nairobi performed eye surgery to close the punctures in the front part of my eyes, and splinted my left arm, which had been dislocated at the elbow. I'm sure they also removed many shrapnel fragments from all over my body.

I soon found myself on a military plane with some of the other embassy employees. Someone said we were being evacuated to Landstuhl, Germany. I remember thinking about the many hours my husband and I had spent in the Landstuhl Hospital when we were stationed in nearby Zweibruecken during Don's military career.

I was so sedated at the time that I really didn't think about what my husband must have gone through when he learned I had been in the embassy at the time of the bombing. He told me later that he assumed I had been out working on the deal for the new office. He was as concerned as anyone else when he saw reports of the incident, but he never imagined I had been a victim.

When he received a call following the embassy attack, he was told his wife suffered lacerations to her face and abdomen and a broken arm. Those injuries didn't sound all that bad, so he wasn't particularly worried—until he saw me in Landstuhl two days after the bombing. In the first moment, he realized that what he had been told gave new meaning to the term "understatement." He told me (much later) that I looked like a "blow-torched raw turkey that had been sprayed with birdshot." My tough, ex-military husband nearly passed out when he first beheld my face. The chaplain on duty in the hospital later apologized to Don for not being there to support him. He said, "No one should have to see what you saw without compassionate preparation."

I'm glad I was unconscious at the time.

Doctors operated on me all day Sunday and into the night. And I'm told we left Germany for the United States in a C-141 at about two o'clock Monday morning.

I remember landing at Andrews Air Force Base for transport to Walter Reed Army Medical Center. I could hear a siren and asked if we were in a hurry. My immediate thought was that I had developed some complication, and could feel anxiety and fear starting to envelop me once more. Don held my hand and reassured me that the driver was just trying to get us through traffic.

At Walter Reed, we were rushed into the emergency room, with the sound of excited voices all around. They let Don stay, which kept me calm and reasonably relaxed. For the next week, Don became my memory, as I drifted in and out of consciousness.

Once settled into the hospital, Danny DeVito, my supervisor from the Department of Commerce, loaned my husband a laptop so he could update family and friends via e-mail. The address list grew to somewhere around two hundred names, and we were told that Don's e-mails were posted on embassy and consulate bulletin boards around the world.

I was flattered and humbled later when one of the consulate drivers told me he had prayed to Allah for me, and he knew I would get through this because I was a good person and had a pure heart. Special blessings like this came in from all over the world and gave me strength to get through the difficult days that lay ahead.

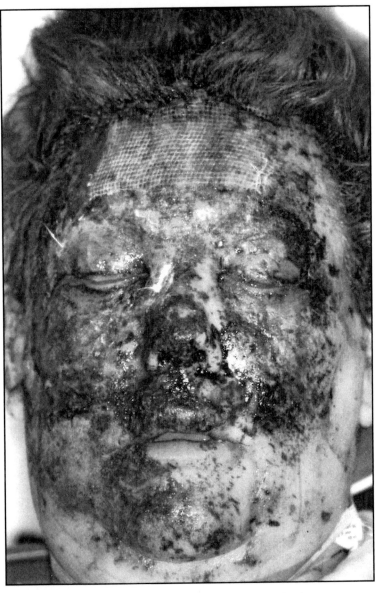

Ellen's arrival photo at Walter Reed Army Medical Center
(You should have seen it in color!)

CHAPTER 5

SURVIVOR

MY FIRST WEEK at Walter Reed was a blur; I was sedated for most of it, so perhaps a fuzzy memory isn't surprising. I do, however, remember being aware of the kindness and gentleness of the doctors and nurses there. I felt so blessed to be at a hospital with a staff that not only ministered to my body, but to my spirit as well.

Don, too, was very attentive. I'm so grateful he stayed by my side as much as the medical team allowed. In fact, as I learned later, he faithfully sat beside me from seven in the morning until eight at night, day after day. What follows is his account of those long days, and then my recollection:

Week 1

Immediately after our arrival on Monday, Ellen was subjected to about seven hours of examination by ophthalmology, reconstructive surgery, orthopedic, and emergency teams. She then underwent eight hours of intensive eye surgery to repair (again) the leaks in both eyes and to remove embedded glass, trash, cinderblock fragments, and any other foreign matter.

She spent the next day and a half in surgical intensive care, where she remained sedated most of that time. While she was there, the plastic surgery team scoured her face to remove the burned skin. The swelling remained, but she looked so much better!

By Wednesday, Ellen's color had improved, the swelling had gone down, and she was able to speak more clearly and coherently. That day her hospital room seemed to have a revolving door. We barely had time to process the information from one doctor or medical team before another one would come in.

Two of the senior ophthalmologists—Dr. Hollifield for the retina and Dr. Trudo for the cornea—consulted with us and gave us a bit more detail on the extent of Ellen's eye injuries. They explained the repairs they had made and told us about a larger problem. The lenses in both eyes had clouded, so, although they could see with ultrasound that there was still foreign matter in the eyes, they couldn't see through the lens to the retina to assess the damage. At this point we weren't really sure what that meant for the long term, but we knew we were in capable hands.

I was truly astounded at Ellen's spirits during this time. She laughed and joked and was so grateful to be alive. She even seemed to accept that she might lose some or all of her vision permanently.

On Thursday, we were honored by a visit from U.S. Secretary of Commerce William Daley, and Under Secretary of Commerce for International Trade David Aaron. The men expressed their concern, thanked her for her service, and encouraged her to persevere in her recovery. It was the high point of Ellen's day.

Friday brought yet another important visitor. Secretary of State Madeleine Albright stopped in to see the Nairobi patients. She was extremely gracious and spoke with Ellen and me for several minutes. Ms. Albright held Ellen's hand and told her to call if she needed any sort of help. She left with tears in her eyes.

Ellen's eye surgery scheduled for this week was postponed, and we were told to expect anywhere from two to six more eye surgeries over the next several weeks or months. The doctors were pleased with how the eyes were healing, but we didn't have a clear prognosis or timeframe. We were, however, committed to doing everything we could to restore her vision and heal her body.

When I arrived at Walter Reed, I was given the name "Miss Gloria" to protect my identity. All Nairobi patients were given "code names" to protect us from possible further attacks and the news media. Major Hyacinth Joseph was the head nurse on Ward Six, and she made certain that our safety and privacy were second only to our healing.

As "Miss Gloria," I led a life I never could have imagined. Every day Don would help me into a wheelchair, and we'd make our way down the long hall to the ophthalmologist's office. I had to gear up mentally for these exams, because the doctor would have to force my eyelids open. One of them, dear Captain Hutchun, was so gentle (but her hands were very cold!), and would always encourage me, saying, "Okay,

Ellen, we can do this." The pain was so intense it made me whimper like a child. Those exams seemed to last forever, but according to Don, they only lasted about ten minutes.

I could feel the heavy scab—caused from the debris of the building and blood—that etched itself from the crown of my head around my forehead and over to my right earlobe. It felt so awful and thick, itched like crazy, and I couldn't reach it to scratch it. Finally, I just couldn't stand it anymore. I asked one of the nurses to wash my hair, so she brought a basin to the end of the bed. As I held my head over the water, she gently peeled away the layers of pulverized cement and glass, blood and other body fluids. It took several sessions to remove the scab completely, and we found there was actually a hole on the top of my head right down to my skull.

At night, after Don left, I would lie in bed, my mind obsessing as I deliberated the future: *I'm useless now; there's nothing I can do; no one would want to have a blind person around. I'll never work again. Maybe I can sit in the hospital nursery and rock the babies. I don't need to see to do that.* I thought about all the material possessions I had amassed in Saudi Arabia; they were now totally worthless to me. I thought about the little ranch we had bought in Texas. I didn't see how we could ever live there, because I was terrified of stepping out into the black nothingness around me. Grasping at my shred of hope in God, I would pray the rosary, and drift off to sleep.

Week 2

On Tuesday Ellen was able to detect close finger movement with her left eye as well as the ophthalmologist's flashlight with both eyes, which was a great sign.

She had been complaining of pain in her upper right thigh. As it turned out, a piece of metal about one centimeter by a half centimeter was lodged in there. It was several inches from the entrance wound, so no wonder it was sore! Surgeons wouldn't typically operate without first pinpointing the exact location of the fragment. But that would require an MRI, and Ellen couldn't (and still can't) have an MRI because of all the other metal fragments in her body. The procedure could cause more damage than the fragments themselves.

We also found out that Ellen had perforations of both eardrums. The left one wasn't too serious, but the right one would likely require surgery in a month or two.

When Don returned to his hotel that evening, I wrestled with my fear that someone was out to get me and that they'd actually find me. Even though I knew the terrorists hadn't been after me personally, I wondered if they would look for those who had been injured, and try to finish what the bombs had started. Hoping to distract myself, I asked Lt. Haynes, one of the nurses, for a radio, and she tuned it to a local Christian station. This dear, sweet angel of mercy would also come into my room at night when things were quiet and pray with me, especially before upcoming surgery. Those prayers meant a lot to me.

Once I began to relax, I heard a knock at my door. The visitor identified himself as Sergeant Meany (he was anything but that) who asked what he could do for me. I was grateful for the company and told him I'd appreciate it if he would just sit and talk with me. So he did. As I remember, he said that he was a nurse on one of the wards and that he was stationed in Dhahran during Desert Storm. He helped with the survivors of a Scud missile attack when one exploded near a tent full of American soldiers.

As the conversation moved from war to football to politics, I felt safe enough to drift off to sleep. I never heard from him again, and sometimes I wonder if God didn't just send an angel that night to calm my fears.

On Wednesday we spent quite a while listening to the eye surgeon explain what he was going to do for Ellen's left eye the following day.

He told us the surgery would take anywhere from two to twelve hours, and there was a possibility that they'd have to remove the lens, replacing it at a later date, and also the cornea, replacing it at the end of the operation. Though he couldn't say what her vision would be like after the surgery, he was confident he would at least be able to assess the extent of the damage to the retina.

Ellen had many visitors that day, which helped take her mind off the impending surgery. Two dear friends from the Jeddah Consulate, Hala Buck and Candy Tietjen, stopped by for moral support. Some of Ellen's friends from the Nairobi Embassy, Gus Maffery and Susan Wiley, also came to see us. Susan was in Ellen's office just minutes before the explosion, and she and Ellen were discussing what a "soft target" the embassy was. She had gone back to her office to drop off the copies, leaving the building. She was about two miles away when she felt the explosion. Thank God, she escaped without a scratch.

Last, but not least, Senator Bob Dole visited for a while with an offer of support. He also left with tears in his eyes.

Before leaving that night, Ellen told me she believed God had a purpose for her, or she wouldn't have been spared. If God grants her sight, she told me, she will be grateful. If He does not, she will be grateful that she is alive to fulfill His purpose. Prior to this time I was probably closer to being an agnostic than a Christian. Although I attended Sunday school and church from infancy to age eighteen, when I joined the army, I would not describe myself as a godly person at that time in my life. I did pray occasionally, "just in case," I guess; but my heart didn't belong to the Lord. However, it was then that I started to really believe and began to pray. She was alive and shouldn't have been. She had been spared for me and for whatever purpose God had in mind for her.

Thursday morning Ellen went into surgery for her left eye at 9:35 A.M. Dr. Trudo talked to me at about 6:15 P.M. in the evening to tell me she was still in surgery for her retina with Dr. Hollifield, and that it would likely take several more hours to complete the operation.

They found at least one tear in the inside wall that had not been previously seen, plus several pieces of glass embedded in the walls of the eye. Each problem had to be repaired before they could proceed to the next step.

At the conclusion of the operation, the doctors told me they were pleased with the repairs they'd made. However, due to the extensive damage to the eye, it would be six weeks or so before Ellen could start "seeing" with that eye. They had placed an air bubble in her eye that would slowly be displaced by the natural fluid the body produces. When that process was complete, the doctors would be able to test her sight.

Ellen said John spoke to her in a dream and told her she would see again. I took that as a good sign.

On Sunday, only three days after her surgery, the doctor expressed concern about Ellen's right eye, which was still inflamed and wouldn't improve until the glass and other objects were removed. We elected to schedule the operation for the right eye the following day. Although this surgery wouldn't take as long, the lens would need to be removed and the cornea replaced.

We were so grateful for good Samaritans who take time to fill out organ donor cards. Cornea donors offer hope to those who have lost their sight, such as my wife.

Week 3

Ellen's surgery went as well as expected, and the doctors anticipated a positive outcome. However, as with the previous surgery, the results would not be available for several weeks.

As the days went by, she grew stronger and more able to get around. This week she took her longest walk since Nairobi—sixty yards.

By Thursday she began complaining of headaches. The doctors found no sign of infection or any other cause, which was frustrating to Ellen, who was in quite a bit of pain.

A team of ophthalmologists examined Ellen's eyes each day. They were all very happy with Ellen's progress and seemed almost amazed that she was responding to the surgeries and treatment so well.

Week 4

Ellen's headaches weren't improving. An injection would relieve the pain for several hours, but often it would return as soon as the medicine wore off.

On Wednesday she saw a neurologist, who did several motor-function tests and ordered a complete CT scan. At this point, the best he could tell us was that post-traumatic headaches are very common in cases such as this.

Friday brought the best news we'd heard in quite a while: Ellen could leave the hospital! After almost a month, she had a pass for Labor Day weekend. I received training in administering her fifteen or so medications (most to the eyes), and it looked to be a full-time job. But I didn't care. I was just so happy to have her with me again; I could deal with the rest.

I was looking forward to leaving the hospital, as well. Up until this time, I had only walked around inside or on the grounds.

Riding the shuttle was a scary ordeal for me, but that was nothing compared to the terror I felt when I had to take that first step down onto the street from the bus. I was stepping into nothingness; I couldn't see the ground. For all I knew, there *was* no ground! When I could see, I had never really considered how much I relied on my vision to orient myself to my surroundings—and how secure I felt within that orientation. Now I could sense no physical boundaries—just empty space. I had to force myself to take that step, to believe that the blackness engulfing me at the moment wasn't going to swallow me completely. But I stepped out and it was okay. What a relief!

Saturday night, Don received an e-mail from Danny DeVito, my former supervisor. Danny had gone back to the U.S. Nairobi Embassy for the first time that week. What follows is his report of the damage:

> I have no idea how Ellen and Tobias survived. There is only one other person I know that was working in an office on the backside of the embassy that survived—and that is Caroline in Personnel. The damage to the offices is incredible. The reinforced block walls that separated the SCO Office from Priscah and Ellen's office and also between Priscah and Ellen's office, and Adam and Tobias' office were just completely blown out as if they were made of papier-mâché. Even the wall separating our offices from the hallway was destroyed; and it knocked down the wall on the other side of the hallway.
>
> I guess for Ellen to be able to conceptualize it, there was someone in the men's bathroom at the time the blast occurred. He was hurt (badly bruised) by the wall that blew in on him. For that wall to crumble, the blast first had to pass through two other cement block walls.
>
> One of the best examples of the force of the blast that allowed me to conceive of it was when I read about cars on the street in front of the Co-Op Bank (about forty yards from the car bomb), which were picked up and thrown against buses that were stopped on the other side of the street picking up passengers.

By this time, several people had told us that my experience and resolve had increased their faith. Hearing this report made me realize even more that God was with me and had saved my life for a purpose.

Week 5

Tuesday brought some great news: Ellen was able to detect hand motion in both eyes, up and down and back and forth. That was a big first step! The doctors ordered a pair of glasses for her with +9 lenses (Coke bottles) and an additional +2.5 bifocal. This was a temporary replacement for the lenses they removed from the inside of her eyes. As the gas bubble got smaller in each eye, the doctors were hoping she would be able to see around the bubble. At that point, they would be able to do a partial assessment of her sight. We still didn't know what the future held, but all signs were still good.

Week 6

Last week the ophthalmologists told us Ellen didn't need to be seen for a few days, so she didn't have an eye exam until Wednesday. Ellen again detected motion and direction of motion with her right eye, but only motion with her left eye. However, she was also able to count the right number of fingers two out of three times! This was still with no lenses in her eyes and no glasses. In retrospect, these milestones seem so small, yet they were major events in our lives at the time.

Also this week, Ellen got her voice back. Since the fifteen-hour operation on her left eye, her voice had been very thin and difficult to hear—probably because of the respirator tube that was down her windpipe for almost a day and a half. She had told me before that it seemed as though her mouth, tongue, and lips were "separate," but now they feel as though they're back "together" again.

Week 7

Ellen's mother and brothers arrived for a visit; it was so good to have family and friends around at times like this.

We saw Dr. Hollifield, the retina specialist, and his staff this week, and though they said recovery is progressing better than they expected, we still didn't know how much sight Ellen would regain. It would be months before all the operations were completed and the eyes would be healed.

Our Eritrean housekeeper and dear friend, Tseghe (pronounced Tseegay), who had worked for us for five years in Jeddah, arrived this week. She began as our housekeeper, and then grew to be a confidant and friend. She is a very godly person and we love her as a daughter. Tseghe was about five foot one inch, size ten, about 130 pounds and very pretty. She is very well mannered, and was raised in an Italian Catholic girls' day school. When war broke out in her country, she was married with two children, and elected to go to Saudi Arabia to earn money to send back to her family. Her children were raised by her mother, since her husband had left them for another woman. She would take care of Ellen when I went back to work in Saudi Arabia. I knew she'd be a great help and comfort to Ellen when I was gone.

This week Dr. Trudo declared the cornea transplant officially healed. Additional good news: During the last exam Ellen quickly and accurately counted fingers with her left eye. This was the first time for counting with her "bad" eye! Of course, she couldn't actually "see" yet. Her eyes were still closed all day (except for "eyelid" exercises), and she had no internal lens in either eye. She could only count the fuzzy outline of fingers at certain angles and distance, but even that was real progress for the level of damage she had. With all the ground she was gaining, she was still blind. However, these good signs gave us hope that she would eventually have some level of vision—perhaps nearly normal in "at least one eye." Only time would tell.

Ellen's eardrum surgery was scheduled for the following week. While she was under, the eye surgeons would take the opportunity to make any adjustments to the air bubbles, trim the corneal stitches, and whatever else they saw that needed tweaking. Other surgeons would remove a number of small pieces of glass that were still coming out of her face and upper body. She could often pick them out herself as they came to the surface (that continues to this day), but some stayed just below the surface and would cause pain whenever she bumped the affected body part.

Week 8

Ellen went into surgery around noon. Dr. Elizabeth Blair, the Ear, Nose, and Throat specialist (ENT), repaired the right eardrum and patched the left eardrum, removing a couple of small pieces of glass from Ellen's neck that were on the surface.

Ellen had complained for more than a month about a pain in the back of her right thigh. The doctors all assumed she had a shard of glass embedded there, because it didn't show up on X-ray. But when the Dr. Blair went fishing for it, she removed a 3½-inch piece of wood about 5/16 inch wide on one end and sort of pointed on the other end. This piece of wood apparently entered at the top front of Ellen's thigh and was removed on the bottom left side about four inches above her knee. Dr. Blair was thereafter known as the "Ear, Nose, and Thigh" doctor throughout the hospital.

After Dr. Blair completed her work, the ophthalmologists began theirs. The results were a mixed bag. The good news was that the retina in the left eye was still okay. The bad news was that the retina in the right eye had partially detached. The surgeon told me it was probably due to the scars in the wall of the eye "pulling" as they formed. Also, the cornea in the right eye was still swollen, which was not good, but it was still clear and there were no signs of rejection.

During the previous two surgeries, the doctors had put Scleral Buckles around each eye. This is a plastic device that helps prevent retina detachments. The buckle is positioned between the eyeball and the membrane that surrounds the eye (the conjunctiva). The conjunctiva was sewn over the buckle when it was placed around the eye. During this most recent surgery the doctors noted that the buckle was exposed in both eyes. This may have been due to a breakdown of the conjunctiva caused by the heat of the explosion or chemical contamination from it. They put

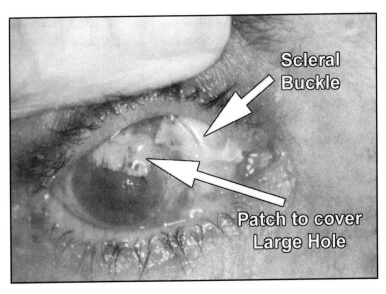

Right eye showing Scleral Buckle and patch covering a large hole.

patches over all exposed parts, and we would just have to watch and wait.

I was not released from Walter Reed, but I was able to stay in our suite at the Malonge House, which is a residential facility for family and outpatients at Walter Reed. Even though we had expected it, when word came that Don would have to return on November 7 to his logistics job in Saudi Arabia where he worked on an air defense contract, I crumbled emotionally. I was terrified of being left on my own, and cried every night. Tseghe would hold me and tell me, "It's going to be okay; you can do this." Tseghe was such a comfort to me. She soothed my fears, bathed me, fed me, and loved me. Her encouragement and steadfastness bolstered me when I felt low, and she never allowed me to forget to be thankful for all the good things I still had in my life.

Being blind brought so many changes, and one that I hadn't really anticipated was the fact that I was always "in my head." Without any visual distractions, I felt trapped with my thoughts and feelings and fears. I hadn't realized how simply seeing familiar faces and objects helps to anchor our minds and emotions, shifting us away from self.

I knew I couldn't live enclosed in my own dark world for the rest of my life, so I determined to find more support. My search started with Columbia Lighthouse for the Blind in Washington, D.C. I was impressed with their progressive ideas and opportunities, but their office was located in a pretty tough part of town. I didn't think I would feel safe going there without Don once he was back in Saudi Arabia.

We heard about a Department of Commerce employee that was blind, and arranged to visit him at his office. He amazed me! His computer talked to him, both speaking every letter that he typed, and then reading everything that was on the screen. The software was a program called "JAWS for Windows." He gave me hope that I might return to doing my job, even if I did not regain my sight. He understood my concerns about the location of the Columbia Lighthouse, and suggested we try Volunteers for the Visually Handicapped (VVH).

When we returned to our hotel, I called VVH and made an appointment. We met with Gail Snider a day or so later, and I told her that I wanted to learn how to live as a blind person.

"You need to talk with my ex-husband, Harold Snider," she said as she dialed his number. I spoke to him and explained again what I desired.

"Sure! I'd be happy to help you," he said. "When can I come and visit with you?"

"What? You mean—now?"

"I can be there in an hour."

True to his word, Harold, who is blind, along with his sighted wife, knocked on our hotel room door less than sixty minutes later.

They sat down and Harold began asking questions. How did I perceive my life would be different now that I was blind? What did I want him to do for me?

As I tried my best to answer, I was so distracted by his cell phone. I could hear the "beep-beep" of the key pad as he entered numbers, calling one person after another. I thought his fingers must have been flying! When I asked a question about blind school, he immediately called JoAnn Wilson, director of the Louisiana Center for the Blind (LCB). When I told him I liked to cook, he immediately called Barbara, a blind gourmet cook in Missouri. I had never considered whether a blind person could do such a thing—and do it so proficiently.

Our time together filled me with bright hope and a new perspective on what opportunities lay ahead.

Harold and Tseghe were both godsends at this time in my life, especially with Don back in Saudi Arabia. Harold motivated me, and Tseghe watched out for me. Yet one other person came alongside and provided invaluable assistance as well. That was my mobility instructor from Volunteers for the Visually Handicapped, Donna Sauerberger, who was determined to help me face and conquer certain fears. She came once a week to my hotel to show me how to use the long white cane. I remember the first time I had to go down the steps. I was so terrified; I tried to go down on my hands and knees! But she admonished me, "Get up! Is that what you would you do if there was a fire? How would you get out?"

She took me to the fire escape for the first several lessons. I would feel the steps with my long white cane, hold on to the handrail with my other hand, and slowly descend and ascend.

The next session took us to the hotel lobby, which had a double staircase from the ground floor to the mezzanine. I would go up the right stairs and down the left stairs with my long white cane. Up and down, up and down—for an hour and a half! When I was done, I felt as though I had scaled Mount Everest and planted a flag. I had mastered the stairs—and my fear.

Of course, as every climber knows, there's always another peak, always another mountain range. Once I got the hang of getting around the hotel, we proceeded to the great outdoors. We walked out the front door, went about two blocks, and made our way back.

At this time I also started learning Braille, which was made more difficult by the numbness in the fingers of my right hand caused by nerve damage during my most recent surgery. Besides Braille, I received instruction on how to use my computer again. I was a self-taught typist and always looked at the keyboard as I typed. I had to practically start from scratch learning key positions, but I finally learned to type. My computer is "voice enabled," as well, so whatever a sighted person is able to see on the screen is read to me by JAWS. This includes everything I type. Hearing my mistakes aloud is good motivation for correcting them!

I struggled to accept the long white cane. I had a hard time believing the cane would actually get me where I wanted to go, or that the cane could actually be my eyes. I wasn't all that thrilled about learning Braille, either. I was a reluctant student at first, and often thought, *Why do I need to learn this when I'm not going to stay blind?*

November 1998

In November, I had the Scleral Buckle removed from my left eye. It had accomplished what the doctors hoped it would, and they informed me that to leave it in place would eventually cause more problems than solve. They told me that it would still be about six months before I would know exactly how much vision I would have in the end.

At another appointment, the cornea specialist told me he knew of no case where someone sustained the eye injuries as severe as mine and retained their eyes; that I was pushing the frontier of medical research and repair for eye injuries.

I had much to be grateful for that Thanksgiving, including the very gracious Dolly Harrod from the International Trade Agency in the Commerce Department. She knew Don was out of the country, so she and her family invited Tseghe and me to join them for the holiday.

Just before Thanksgiving, I received word that I, along with several others, would be receiving a gold medal from the United States government on December tenth. It didn't take long for me to start worrying about the logistics of the ceremony: How would I make my way to the stage? Find the steps? How would I keep from falling on my face? How would I receive the medal from the Secretary of Commerce? How would I get back to my seat?

These concerns were minor, however, compared to the larger question of my employment. I received a great deal of personal satisfaction and affirmation from my work, and I wasn't willing to give that up. I felt so vulnerable not knowing what the future held regarding my job. I also wasn't sure who was going to pay for medical expenses I would likely incur in the months and years ahead. I wanted reassurance from the Department of State that my medical needs would be taken care of. At that point, however, I was simply grateful that the Department of Labor paid Tseghe to be my non-medical attendant, which enabled her to stay in Washington, D.C., and care for me. With Don back in Saudi Arabia, I don't know what I would have done without her.

December 1998

Don arrived back in Washington, D.C., in early December to attend the award ceremony. After being apart for a month, it was wonderful to hear his voice undistorted by phone connections, hold his hand, and feel the love and support that emanated from his embrace.

A few days later, we attended the ceremony. Since I had no clothes with me, I borrowed a dress to wear to the ceremony. I was one of thirty-five gold and seventy-eight silver medal recipients. Of course, all my fears proved to be unfounded (as most fears are). When my name was called, I was escorted to the stage by August ("Gus") Maffrey, Commercial Attaché in Nairobi at the time of the bombing. (Gus had left the Nairobi embassy only moments before the attack. Had he been in his office at the time of the explosion, he would have most likely been killed.) As I carefully climbed the steps, someone took hold of my hand, guiding me over to the Secretary of Commerce, who embraced me and gave me the award. I stood there for awhile before being escorted from the stage. Don informed me later that I had received a standing ovation that went on for almost two minutes. I was overwhelmed by the applause and humbled by the care expressed by all these people I didn't even know.

The awards ceremony was truly a highlight in my life, but the next day brought even more excitement.

At my ophthalmologist appointment, I put on my new sixteen-power glasses, and the doctor asked me to try to read what was on a piece of paper he held about five feet away, with my right eye covered.

"Seven," I told him. I could hardly contain myself. I could see it!

He continued the exercise by reducing the print size, and I could see down to about two-inch letters with both eyes.

That night, while Don and I were watching TV, I said, "I can see my fingers. I can probably crochet." I put on my glasses, and I could even read a one-inch headline in the newspaper. Even though I was still "legally blind," we were both so thankful to God for this exciting development.

Don returned to Saudi Arabia just before Christmas, and Tseghe and I accepted my Cousin Tina's invitation to spend the holiday with her family in Doylestown, Pennsylvania. Our only problem was how to get there. We decided to take the train, and my cousin agreed to meet us at the station.

This trip was another new experience, and I struggled to contain my fear. I remember sitting alone on a bench while Tseghe left me to get a newspaper. I remember thinking, *If someone tries to steal my purse, I can't do a thing to stop him.* I felt so vulnerable!

Fortunately, the train ride was uneventful and even pleasant. We spent three wonderful days with my family and weren't particularly looking forward to returning to Walter Reed. However, our spirits were refreshed and replenished, and Tseghe and I were ready to face whatever lay ahead.

On the twenty-eighth of December, I had my first facial laser treatment to remove the "tattooing" from the bombing. Residue from the explosion had penetrated my face, leaving it blue and looking as if I'd been inked by a drunken tattoo artist. The treatment I received was much like a deep chemical peel, and removed about 60 percent of the markings.

As a belated Christmas gift, my son, Michael, along with his wife, Shannon, and my grandson Andrew, came to

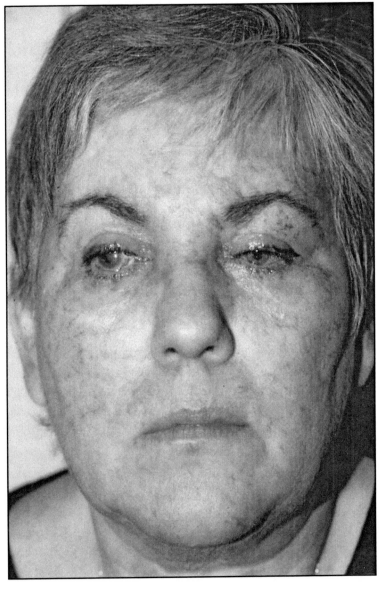

Blast tattooing on Ellen's face before laser surgery

Washington, D. C., to see me. The visit was filled with firsts: This was the first time Michael had seen me face to face since the bombing; both Michael and Tseghe visited the White House for the first time; and best of all, four-year-old Andrew played in the snow for the first time. What refreshment to my soul to hear his shouts of delight and joyous laughter.

The holidays passed quickly, filled with visits from family and many friends, old and new. I missed Don terribly, however. So when I asked about a reunion, my doctors told me that if everything checked out to their satisfaction at my next appointment, I would be cleared to move back to Saudi Arabia for several weeks.

January 1999

A few days before I was to leave for "home" in Saudi Arabia, I noticed a lump on my abdomen—and it had nothing to do with my trepidation about flying blind for the first time. Tseghe took me to the emergency room, where X-rays were taken. I was still carrying around quite a bit of metal shrapnel, and one of the sites had become infected. I was getting used to the idea of being a repository of various types of scrap material, so I wasn't particularly upset. A surgeon made a two-inch incision, cleaned out the infection, patched me up, and I was on my way a few hours later.

On January twelfth, Tseghe and I took a cab to the airport to return to Saudi Arabia. We were both nervous and excited about the trip. Tseghe is reasonably fluent in English, but her accent can still make it difficult for people to understand her. Because of this, the cab driver took us to the wrong gate. When we checked with the airline representative, he said we were in the wrong terminal and that we had to go another building two blocks away. I got upset and started crying. Fortunately, a Good Samaritan offered to help. He got a cab to take us to the right gate. Under duress, we finally made it.

The flight was uneventful and long! I was so impatient to be with Don again. Tseghe was a godsend, but my husband is my rock. And at that time, I still felt somewhat vulnerable and unsure of myself. With him by my side, however, I felt strong and confident, certain that together we could meet whatever challenge lay in our path.

Back at the house, I reveled in being home. Remember, I'd spent the last five months in hospital and hotel rooms. It felt so good just to be surrounded by familiar and comfortable "stuff."

Toward the end of January, Maria, a friend who was married to one of the consulate employees, asked me if I wanted to join a writers' workshop. I'd been toying with the idea of writing a book about this ordeal, so I accompanied her to a meeting. The people there were so welcoming; I attended every week until returning to Washington.

February 1999

Medically speaking, February was a "maintenance" month for me. I still had regular checkups with eye specialists, now at the El-Maghraby Eye Hospital, and with other doctors at the Al-Salama Hospital, one of the newest and most modern medical facilities in that part of the world. These prominent doctors treated me with kindness and respect, and to our amazement, we were never charged for the world-class care I received. The doctors concurred that I was doing very well considering the amount of damage I had sustained, and they praised the great work performed by the Walter Reed Army Medical Center staff. I was blessed to have great care from dedicated, conscientious medical professionals wherever I went for treatment.

Ellen stayed pretty busy every day. She went to her office once a week to help sort out things that had been in limbo when the bombing happened.

Friends visited frequently; they read to her or helped her go through the house, deciding what needed to be thrown out, sold, or shipped home when we left. Each afternoon a friend came to take Ellen and Bobbi, our dog, for a walk around the compound. And she even shopped with friends. Although many things had changed, one of Ellen's habits remained unaffected by her experience. If she said she would be home by eight o'clock, I was to interpret that as "sometime before midnight." To this day, when Ellen gets into her "shop-till-she-drops" mode, she loses all track of time.

Throughout those months, her attitude about what had occurred continued to amaze me. She did not (and still doesn't) hate Osama bin Laden. She knows in her heart that he will answer to God on his judgment day, so any ill feelings she would have are meaningless and a waste of time and energy. She said, "Being blind isn't too bad, just inconvenient." I, on the other hand, am not quite so forgiving, but I'm trying.

I was invited to speak at the American Ladies of Jeddah monthly meeting to tell them about the bombing, and I accepted with pleasure.

Everyone was very solicitous, and when I finished speaking I could hear sniffles in the room.

One of the ladies told me she had written a poem about my experience when she heard that I would be speaking, and asked if she could read it to the group of one hundred fifty women. Delighted, she let me include it in my book:

Who Did This?

On a quiet Friday morning
When nothing seemed to be awry,
A sudden blast broke the silence
As debris seemed to fall from the sky.

Two buildings started to tumble
And shocked screams filled the air.
For a moment, no one could fathom
What had happened; what a scare!

Even before the dust could settle,
In another country, not far away,
Tanzania felt the rumble as
Another bomb disrupted their day.

This deed was orchestrated,
Like a "secret" plan somehow.
It was not just a random act
It was planned; we know that now.

These bombs were meant to hurt, to kill,
And cause much grief and pain;
It woke us up as we realized
Terrorism had struck again.

Nairobi, Kenya, is a place
That no one would dare suspect
That terror loomed as someone planned
To make this place a wreck.

And we all know there was a plan.
Someone wanted to hit and not miss;
We wonder as we look in shock
And ask, *Who did this?*

—Bessie M. Campbell

On one visit to the consulate office, the driver who picked me up asked me how I was doing. He told me he and his co-workers had been praying for me, that I was a good person, and that he was so sorry for what had happened. He believed Allah would help me to get better. I was so humbled that he would even think of me, and I was reminded again that the actions of the few seldom represent the beliefs of the majority.

March 1999

Shortly before Tseghe and I returned to Washington, D.C., and Walter Reed, I had my eyes checked one last time. Dr. Al-Maghraby and his staff at the eye hospital told us the retina was still in place in both eyes; no sign of trouble there. However, both my natural cornea in the right eye and the graft in the left eye were cloudy, likely requiring replacement.

We also finally got up the nerve to have my vision tested. The news wasn't as good as we had hoped: Corrected vision in both eyes was less than 20/400 (20/200 is legally blind). However, the doctors at Walter Reed had indicated that they could do some medical magic, so we anticipated more improvement.

On March 21, we left for the United States. As much as I was looking forward to possibly improving my vision with the help of doctors at Walter Reed, it was still difficult to say good-bye to our Jeddah friends. We had been loved and blessed by many, and even now we look back at that time in our lives with gratitude for the people God brought across our path.

April/May 1999

My first eye exam back at Walter Reed went very well. The doctors were pleased with my progress, although my eyes still had a lot of healing to do. Their prognosis was always "cautiously optimistic," which means they really didn't know. But I held on to those words; they gave me hope. They did not schedule any procedures, and said they would not need to see me again until July. Photos were also taken of my eyes—both internal and external—to use in training at Walter Reed.

In the meantime, I would continue my life as a blind person, doing what I needed to do to learn how to live this way. So while holding onto this hope for sight, I reluctantly proceeded, step by step, into an unforeseen future without it.

If I thought dealing with blindness, ear infections, and shrapnel all over my body was bad enough, I was wrong. I contracted shingles, an excruciatingly painful viral infection of the nerves. The bug that causes it is the same as chicken pox. It can occur in various places on the body, and I had it around my torso. Fortunately, the rash started to itch after a few days, which meant the infection would soon recede. I had never welcomed itchy skin before, but since it indicated the end of this particular ordeal, I was more than happy to accept the comparatively minor discomfort.

April also brought more shrapnel removal and another laser treatment for my face—nothing compared to the agony of shingles!

Don soon returned to Jeddah, and a week after that I said good-bye to Tseghe as well. Since I would soon be enrolled at the Louisiana Center for the Blind, I wouldn't need her as a paid assistant any longer. Her visa would expire soon, so with my blessing, she would spend her last few months in the States with her sister in Seattle.

After a weeklong visit with my sister-in-law, Trish, in San Antonio, Texas, she and I flew to Washington, D.C., where I would attend a conference, sponsored by the Department of State, for victims of the Nairobi and Tanzania terrorist attacks. This would be the first time since the bombings that all of us would be together.

The conference, which featured appearances by Secretary of State Madeline Albright, Attorney General Janet Reno, Under Secretary of Commerce for International Trade David Aaron, and representatives from several other federal agencies, began on May 5, 1999.

The first session opened with an introduction by the admiral who had directed the investigation of the bombings. He told us they had received warnings of a bomb threat prior to August 7, 1998, but it had been discounted as "not credible."

When the speaker asked for questions from the floor, several of the attendees became very vocal and passionate, demanding answers to the unanswerable:

"Why did it take so long for the bodies to be returned?" "Why have we received so little compassion from the people handling our requests for assistance?" And worst of all, "Why are our loved ones dead?"

The heavy load of pain and anguish in the room lay like choking smog over us all. As I sat there listening to my coworkers and their dependents, I could hear grief, anger, and frustration in their voices. I realized how fortunate I was to be unconscious immediately following the bombing. Because of my serious injuries, I hadn't really grasped much of what had transpired the day of the attack.

I tried to offer comfort where I could. At break times, psychologists made themselves available to help people with reliving and recounting their experiences during and after the bombing.

The conference lasted a week, overflowing our brains with information. Much of the time I felt as though I was caught in a flooded ditch, unable to pull myself out of the hurt and pain that swirled around me.

I didn't have much time to dwell on the conference, however. At its conclusion, I found myself on another plane, headed off to yet another new experience. I was on my way to the Louisiana Center for the Blind, one of the National Federation for the Blind (NFB) training centers for the blind, by the blind; meaning mostly blind staff and instructors. As I flew to Louisiana, I hoped the NFB philosophy, *"If a blind person has proper training and opportunity, blindness can be reduced to a physical nuisance,"* would come true for me.

CHAPTER 6

BOOT CAMP FOR THE BLIND

IN MAY 1999, I got off the plane filled with anxiety; I hated traveling by myself. It was Saturday, late in the afternoon.

I found a seat and waited for what seemed like hours. I had thoughts that maybe I had arrived on the wrong day or time, and I wondered what would happen if nobody showed up. (This was before the widespread use of cell phones.)

Finally a man from the Louisiana Center for the Blind (LCB) approached, introduced himself, and apologized for being late. He escorted me to his truck, and we took off for the school, stopping for a fast-food meal along the way.

When we arrived at the school's apartment complex, one of the sighted teachers greeted me and then took me to my apartment. I was shocked. I hadn't expected to be on my own the first night. Without vision, I did not know where to find the sheets and towels, or even the bathroom!

She also introduced me to my mentor, Lawanna, who was also blind. The two of them commenced to help me make my bed to sleep in, somewhat to my relief. Then the sighted teacher asked if I needed to go to Wal-Mart. Well, since the apartment had furniture, but no food or other supplies, the answer to her question seemed obvious. I bit my tongue, accepted her offer, and bought everything I would need to set up housekeeping. When I was finally left alone in my apartment at about eleven thirty that night, I burst into tears. I had never felt so alone in my life. I eventually drifted to sleep, and when I woke up the next morning, I felt a little better.

Lawanna came over the next day to help unpack, and we set about putting the apartment in order, which made me feel a little better. She introduced me to various people, and informed me that on Monday we would go to school. During the first week a van transported us to and from school, but after that, we had to walk the half-mile. I would be on my own once I became familiar with the route.

I was also taken to the office, where I met Neita Ghrigsby. While she asked me questions in order to fill out forms, I began sobbing. *This was it.* I was finally forced to accept the fact that I was blind. I still couldn't see, and I really did not know if that would ever change.

Before I left Neita, she gave me a pair of sleep shades; a mask that covered my eyes and blocked any images or light. At this time I had double vision and I could see shadows, or where light came in from the door or window, but no color. I could see some movement; enough that I did not want to block anything out with sleep shades. The rationale is that if you can function in complete darkness, your confidence will grow. She told me I had to wear the sleep shades all day while classes were in session. That really disheartened me, but Neita probably saved my sanity. To chase away my fears, she gave me a good-morning hug every day for the rest of my stay at LCB.

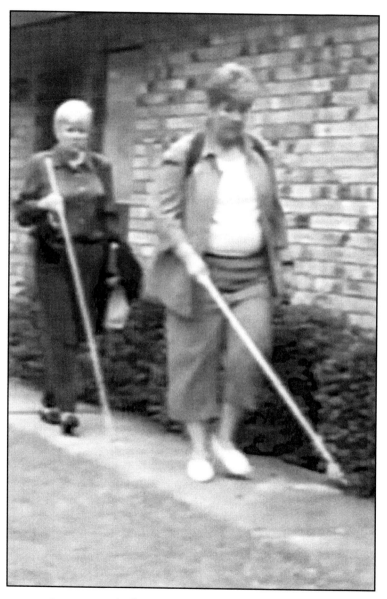

Lawanna and Ellen leaving for classes at LCB – 1999[6]

Lawanna took me to get my schedule, where I cried some more. She told me she would take me to each of my classes that day, and then make sure I got into the van and back to the apartment after school.

My first class was "Mobility," and although I had some cane travel training while at Walter Reed, I was really taught to use my long white cane as my eyes at LCB. That first day's class was pretty traumatic. Roland Allen, my cane travel instructor, took me to a long hall and told me how to walk it, including how to sweep my new "eyes" from side to side. I froze, I was so afraid. I started to cry, but Roland was kind and patient. He told me how he had become blind, which took me out of myself, made me think of someone else. He encouraged me to believe I could get past my fear and learn to get around successfully.

After mobility I had "Braille" with two other students. Jerry Whittle, the Braille instructor, was also pleasant and patient.

From Braille, I went to "Kitchen" with Merilynn Whittle, Jerry's wife, who is sighted. There I would learn to prepare meals from scratch with basic ingredients. Kitchen was a "core" class, which meant I had to pass it before moving on to the next, or graduate from the school.

After Kitchen I had an hour break for lunch, and then Lawanna led me over to the "Wood Shop" where Jerry Darnell, who was sighted, thank God, would try to teach me woodworking using power tools. I could tell it was a big room from the work sounds and echoes. There were sounds of hammering and power tools humming, as well as the smell of fresh varnish. Jerry explained how we would be taught carpentry skills to build confidence. "Just because you're blind doesn't mean you can't do anything," he said. Again, to graduate from the school I would have to build something—a bookcase—anything. I was a bit anxious about shop class to say the least.

Computer class followed shop. After meeting my computer instructor, I didn't feel as intimidated in this class as some of the others. There I received cassettes for an introduction to JAWS, screen reader software for the visually impaired. JAWS allows a blind person to do just about anything on a computer that a sighted person can do.

After computer class I went to my second Mobility class that day. I didn't cry this time.

At the end of the school day, I was exhausted. Finally back at my apartment, I sat down and cried and cried. When I caught my breath, I called my dear friend Harold Snider, in Maryland, and told him how unhappy I was.

"Ellen, this is such a great opportunity. This was just your first day. You'll get more comfortable pretty soon. Don't let it get to you. You'll be okay, I'm sure of it."

I appreciated his encouragement, but I really wanted someone to commiserate with. I was lonely and I hated to be in "Boot Camp for the Blind." So I called Don in Saudi Arabia and we both cried together.

Part of my struggle lay in the fact that this was the first time in my life I was totally on my own—no family, husband, children, colleagues. I was alone, and I didn't like it. I had thought I was so independent, but even the most minor incidents became almost insurmountable obstacles. Dropping a fork on the floor made me sob, as I crawled around on all fours trying to find it. Many nights I would go to sleep praying the rosary and trying to ease my anxiety and fears.

Besides, I didn't really think I belonged there. After all, I had no intention of staying blind, so why should I learn to accept it? Why should I learn to act and function as a blind person when I was going to eventually regain my sight? I felt so trapped! I was here; I had to do what the instructors told me to do, but I absolutely hated it. I saw a therapist for a while, and she helped me through these feelings, but the experience was still really tough.

As the weeks passed, however, I slowly settled into the routine of school. Twice a week we went to the Louisiana Tech College gym after class where I'd walk the track for an hour. When it was time to leave, as long as I accompanied students in and out of the building I was fine, but on the occasion that I was late, I had to find my way out on my own, and it was frustrating.

Wanting to stay in shape but tired of depending on others to get me in and out of the gym, I approached one of the instructors and asked if I could teach water aerobics. I enjoyed taking a class several years before, and felt pretty confident that I could lead a group. Permission was granted, and I taught a class twice a week. Those two hours every week were a bright spot in an extremely difficult time in my life, and they instilled in me a huge feeling of empowerment and self-worth.

I enjoyed my Braille classes, but they were difficult because I did not have good tactile sensation in the fingers on my right hand due to nerve damage during a lengthy operation at Walter Reed. Reading Braille with only my left hand was very slow and exasperating, so I mostly gave up on it, much to the chagrin of Jerry, my instructor.

My Kitchen class gave me a great sense of accomplishment. I actually made biscuits for the first time in my life that did not qualify as doubles for hockey pucks.

Mobility classes were the real challenge, mostly because I was terrified to go out on the street and just let the long white cane be my eyes. As I mentioned, I was required to wear sleep shades, which look basically like a Zorro mask without eye holes. My limited vision was totally blocked out, and it was very hard for me to be in total darkness again.

One of the exercises the instructor liked to assign involved giving each student a different address of a business in town. Within a set amount of time, we would have to find our way using a special compass, and bring back a business card. One day I was on my way to a florist shop when I stepped on an anthill and walked away with a new appreciation for the term "ankle biters." On another day I walked through a fierce storm, which blew my umbrella inside out. Mobility class was definitely a challenge for me.

Around the middle of May my very good friend, Barbara Barton, came to visit for a week. We had formerly met and become good buddies in Saudi Arabia. It was so good to have her at my apartment. We went to movies and restaurants, and even to school together; a good emotional support when I needed it. Thank God for friends.

Shortly after Barbara's visit, video journalists David Snider (Harold's son) and Rolf Behrens came to Ruston, Louisiana, to film a "week in the life of Ellen Bomer," profiling me as a student at the Louisiana Center for the Blind. David and Rolf silently followed me around for several days, capturing my accomplishments and failures. Oh, what a week! No make-up, no "second takes," just real Ellen. One of these days, I hope to see this video.

Don finally returned home from Saudi Arabia in mid June. After a whirlwind ride to Huntsville, Alabama, to drop off our dog, and to Florida to pick up our new car, he came to LCB to spend a few days with me. It was wonderful to be together again. Just holding each other was enough to make our future seem brighter. Unfortunately, his stay was short-lived and he had to return to Huntsville to get our house in order. After nearly ten years of use as a rental property, it was in pretty sad condition.

During the week of July 4, 1999, I met Don in Atlanta where we attended the National Federation for the Blind Annual Convention, a truly amazing event attended by blind people from all over the world. The host hotel that year presented rather challenging logistics for blind people. A huge bank of elevators made it difficult to ascertain which doors were opening at any given moment. The rooms were quite a distance from the main conference hall, and the exhibit area was in a completely different area. After the conference sessions, when we broke to go

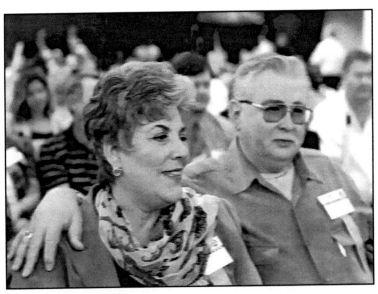

Ellen and Don at NFB Convention - 1999[6]

to workshops, we would hear the simultaneous, nearly deafening sound of approximately two thousand long white canes tap-tapping along the hallways. Thank God for guides provided by the United Parcel Service and the Boy Scouts of America, and also for the Marriott Hotel staff for being so accommodating.

A great highlight of this conference was when NFB President Dr. Mauer asked me to speak. As I addressed the attendees, I told them how astonished I was, upon meeting Dr. Harold Snider and his wife, Linda—over his dexterous use of the cell phone and efficient memory of telephone numbers.

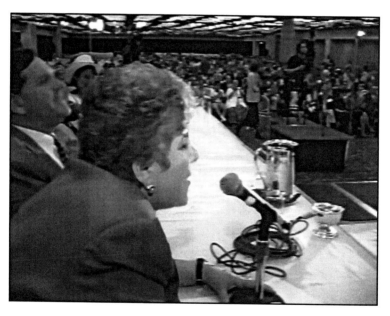

Ellen speaking at NFB Convention – 1999[6]

The conference was fun and inspiring, but I was anxious to get to our Huntsville home for a brief vacation before going back to LCB. Some vacation! Both the bedroom and living room were stacked with boxes from floor to ceiling. I spent the whole week unpacking, not making as much headway as I would have liked. The week flew by, and I was soon back in Louisiana.

CHAPTER 7

ABC NIGHTLINE AND
LCB GRADUATION

WHEN DAVID AND Rolph filmed me in June and July, they had big plans for the finished product. On the first anniversary of the terrorist bombing, which was approaching in August, it was to be featured on ABC's *Nightline*. I would be interviewed at ABC studios in Washington, D.C., along with Harold Snider, by Ted Koppel himself.

———◦∿◦———

As August approached, ABC Television Network press releases promoted two back-to-back programs[1] which were to air August 5 and 6, 1999. They would depict my story of surviving the Nairobi U.S. Embassy bombing and starting life over again as a blind person as chronicled in the film produced by freelance journalists, David Snider and Rolf Behrens—along with extensive interviews, which included promoting Dr. Snider's role as mentor and advocate for the National Center for the Blind.

The broadcast would trace my rehabilitation through LCB and NCB, learning to empower myself with the help of many supporters in the skills of independence—and in gaining a new perspective about life as one now visually impaired.

"I'm kind of like that ship that's slowly being turned. And with each turn and each directional change, I'm getting stronger and stronger and stronger. And I'll be back. It may take me a few more months, but I'll be back," I was quoted.

David Snider, son of a blind father, and the documentary photographer and video journalist, was also quoted in regard to his purpose to bring issues of the blind to a wider audience so that the general public has a better understanding of the effectiveness of their blind "neighbors."

He lives in Washington, D.C., produces The Digital Journalist web site (http://www.digitaljournalist.org), and has been documenting the lives of visually impaired Americans for over ten years.

His partner, Rolf Behrens, is a filmmaker from South Africa who has been operating out of Washington, D.C., for over four years. His work spans Africa as well as South America as producer, cameraman, and editor. He directs the video productions at The Digital Journalist and also teaches the Platypus Workshop.

What an experience it was to be on *Nightline*. After I was escorted from the ABC guest reception studio over to "makeup," Mr. Koppel stopped by to see me while the makeup artist was fussing with my face. With a big smile, he teased me about taking his makeup artist. I'm sure he was just trying to make me more comfortable. And I was pretty impressed that a man of his professional stature applied makeup.

I told him that I had watched his program for many years and followed his daughter's progress as well (a correspondent for CNN), mentioning that he must be very proud of her. He commented that it appeared that she was following in his footsteps. Then we proceeded to the televised set. He was very gracious throughout the interview, and I wasn't as nervous as I thought I would be. At its conclusion, Mr. Koppel asked me what one thing had changed the most in my life since the bombing. I responded with, "I don't eat as much," and he laughed heartily.

An abbreviated description of the Ted Koppel interview with Ellen Bomer and Harold Snider follows:[2]

Thursday, August 5, 1999

As I sat on the studio set across from Ted Koppel, cameras rolling, I told him that in the beginning I had naively grieved over the fact that as a blind person, I wouldn't be able to do anything anymore. I wouldn't be able to see the sky; I wouldn't be able to work; I wouldn't see my husband; I wouldn't see my grandson. I was really scared, and I would go to bed at night crying, and Don would be crying. It was really very traumatic for both of us. And so somewhere toward the end of October 1998, it became evident to both of us that we were going to have to find some support.

Then Dr. Snider and his wife, Linda, came into my and my husband's lives. We were very impressed with them, because they both seemed to be such caring and positive people. And for me it was like, *Wow, he's blind, Linda's sighted, and Don is sighted.* So I felt like this was the family we needed. They would give us the nurturing and support that we really needed to get through this.

Dr. Snider spoke to Mr. Koppel next, reiterating that I seemed like a bamboozled child wandering in the dark at the time, which was exactly how I felt. I was so mesmerized listening to him use his cell phone, that I had hope that I could do it as well.

He went on to tell Mr. Koppel how he had been blind since birth, which never stopped him from being effective as a husband, father, and careerist. And that, as a mentor, he had taught others, as well as myself, new attitudes and basic skills to function as a normal human being.

"Oh, man, it's hard," I commented. "He was the one who suggested I attend Louisiana Center for the Blind to begin my rehabilitation."

I went on to say that when I was first told about Louisiana Center for the Blind, one of the things I was told was that I would be asked to wear sleep shades. And I thought, *How could they take away what little vision that I have? I mean, that must be absolutely horrid.* It wasn't so much the sleep shades as it was "accepting" that I really was blind, and coming to terms with it. But, actually, it's a lot easier to pay attention with sleep shades on than it is without them, because that little bit of vision that you have distracts you.

—◦◦◦—

Ted Koppel asked us to tell him the difference between being one who is newly blind and one who has lifetime blindness.

I said, "I feel like a baby who's learning to walk. I'm learning to crawl first, like a nine-month-old."

Mr. Koppel then asked if I could read a newspaper in Braille, yet.

I answered, "No, sir, I can't. But I can read my name and I can write. I could probably write you a letter in Braille. My instructor would be pleased with that."

He joked that he couldn't read it. And I returned with, "Oh, well, I probably couldn't, either. That's the problem. I can write it, but I can't read it. But I'm learning, and I will conquer it." I did not mention how numbness in my fingers hindered progress.

—◦◦◦—

Both Mr. Koppel and Dr. Snider then kindly expressed sincere admiration over my determination; and I blushed as Dr. Snider extolled me as probably the bravest person he had ever met in his life.

When asked to explain, he said that he had mentored blind people as part of his work with the National

Federation of the Blind for more than thirty years. He started with Vietnam War vets in the sixties when he was in college, and since then with other individuals, and that I had faced my blindness more bravely and more defiantly than the others he had met. And I had done it, to a certain extent, with his help and the help of the members of the National Federation of the Blind.

"Basically, she meets us halfway. That is, she wants to do it. She wants to be all the way back, and that's the big difference."

When Mr. Koppel asked what I meant by the word, *defiant*, I told him I was not going be beaten. "The bombing took away my vision, but it didn't take away me. I'm still here, and I'm still alive, and I'm an American and I'm proud to be an American. That isn't going to change."

I agreed with him that I relied on the fortitude it takes to not let it get me down, defeat me.

"So I have to be true to whatever it is I'm supposed to do. And I figure that if I'm open enough, and I maintain a survivor mentality, someday this bright light's going to go on, and I'm going to know what it is I'm supposed to do."

—◦◦◦—

Mr. Koppel then questioned Dr. Snider about the comfort of sighted people around blind people, not quite sure how sympathetic they need to be, or how helpful.

Dr. Snider answered that he felt that the sighted public, in general, had no expectations of blind people. They don't consider blind people whole, complete human beings, and the training center (LCB), which I was attending, tries to teach its students that, yes, we are whole, complete human beings. The National Federation of the Blind tries to do that at its conventions. People come scared out of their minds, and they leave feeling whole and complete because they went to a convention by themselves, and they could get around and go to the meetings. Basically, it gave them self-confidence. And that's part of what it's about: the desire to change the attitudes of both the blind person and the sighted public to a perspective of confidence.

—◁∧∧∧▷—

When Mr. Koppel asked if I recalled my attitude toward the blind before I became blind myself, I replied, "Yes, I do, and that's part of it. It's difficult to know what's expected of you because I didn't know anyone who was blind before, and all you know is the stereotypes—what you see in movies; what you read in books. I didn't know anyone personally. But [I thought] my eyes are gone now; now I don't have anything. I can't do this; I can't do that; until Harold [Dr. Snider] just walked into that hotel room, saying, 'Yes, you can; yes, you can.'"

—◁∧∧∧▷—

I continued to tell how Joanne Wilson called me from the Center in Louisiana, and asked me what it was I wanted to do that I couldn't do now? And I said I wanted to crochet and I wanted to knit. She replied that I could. And I retorted, "How can I do that? I can't see." And she said, "You don't have to see." That's just part of my rehab, I guess, believing it and making it part of me, because I had sight for fifty-two years. "If we talk about Braille," I told him, "and you tell me to write the word "read," I think in cursive: "r-e-a-d." I do not think in Braille." And so, like I said before, "I'm learning to crawl and then I'll be walking soon, I hope."

⸺⁓⁓⁓⸺

The first day's interview concluded with Ted Koppel asking Dr. Snider to give the audience a sense of what was in store the next day— which would highlight the film showing my educational experience at LCB. He told Mr. Koppel that I was probably a third of the way through my rehabilitation, and that he was confident that I would graduate with flying colors.

Mr. Koppel agreed, and thanked us as he said, "Good night" to our audience.

⸺⁓⁓⁓⸺

Friday, August 6, 1999

Ted Koppel summarized who I was and my experience in the Nairobi U.S. Embassy bombing, which had turned my life upside down and taken away my sight. He finished by saying that the first anniversary of this life-altering event in my life, and the lives of twenty Kenyans who lost their sight—was just a day away. He also remarked that I had shown myself to be a person with "great reserve of courage" during the first part of our interview the previous day.

———⟋⟍⟍⟋———

I began with, "If we touch people . . . then maybe before they throw that bomb or shoot that gun they'll think about what they're doing. I'll be damned if Osama bin Laden beats me. He doesn't know me personally, but he isn't going to beat me and he's not going to defeat me, and I know there are just as many other Americans out there that feel the same way. . . . I have never said anything against Islam. I've always thought it was a beautiful religion, and I don't understand why someone would feel such evil and such hatred for Americans. But I'm determined that that isn't going to defeat me."

———⟋⟍⟍⟋———

Commenting on my "defiant" attitude once again, Mr. Koppel wondered if anger was a necessary part of recovery.

"I think it probably is. I think it's part of the grieving when you lose something," I replied, "whether it's a loved one, your vision, . . . or any appendage. It doesn't consume me, but I feel I'm justifiably angry."

After Mr. Koppel observed that anger also ignited motivation, he asked me to help him understand some of the stages I had gone through in the past year of my recovery.

In response to his request, I told him the first stage was the realization that I was alive, next the gratitude, and then I moved on to how much I hurt and needed to get well. "I don't really think I thought too much about how I felt about anything until maybe October, after all the surgeries."

———ᴧᴧᴧ———

I was medicated most of the time. But after the headaches were gone, when I actually started healing and felt fairly "normal," I wasn't angry.

"I'm only becoming angry, and I'm not really angry, but I'm beginning to stand up for myself and to maybe speak my mind more now. And I believe it's because I don't feel as vulnerable as I did. I've never in my life felt as vulnerable as I did from that blast . . ."

I struggled with qualifying the blast as a "tragedy," when Ted Koppel cut in and confirmed that it was indeed tragic, and did not need to be diminished. He asked me if I ever had moments when I felt like I couldn't continue.

"No," I answered. "I've never thought that, and the reason I haven't . . . is because I know I'm supposed to do it. Whether I like it or not, I know I'm supposed to do it."

———ᴧᴧᴧ———

After a commercial break, Mr. Koppel wanted to focus on living without sight and how the public could understand the blind community better. He asked me if the Department of Commerce was holding my old job for me. I told him yes, but I did not know if I wanted it back. I did want a reason to get up every morning, and had no desire to become a "poster child" for the NFB.

"I would like to motivate people to be nicer to each other, to accept each other for the way they are and not the way they look," I said. Appearances had bottomed-out on my priority list.

When he inquired how my relationships had changed with my husband, friends, and others who have been close to me in the past, I thought carefully and answered.

"I like to think that I'm more—I've always been honest—but I like to think that now I really don't beat around the bush. If someone asks me a question, I give an honest answer. Part of being blind is kind of nice because I can't see your expression. So if I tell you something and you don't particularly like it, I can't tell. So it gives me a little bit more freedom. I wouldn't hurt anyone, but it gives me more freedom."

Mr. Koppel redirected my thought process over to what new impressions I had, if any, of others I had known most of my life, and in the way they treated me. Was it different?

I replied that it was surprising to me that most of my friends had been very supportive and they did not treat me any differently. "They don't hover over me or try to do anything for me. They've accepted me the way I am, and that's really kind of neat because then that kind of says that just because you're blind it doesn't mean that you're not normal."

Upon confessing that his wife was tougher than he was, Ted Koppel asked about my husband's stamina.

"Don's much gentler than I am, but I was still surprised. I think it's because he realized that I almost died and he really wasn't prepared for that. But he's a gentle soul," I related, regarding his unyielding devotion.

—⁂—

Mr. Koppel wanted me to give the audience some road rules for occasions when they may be associating in some capacity with a blind person. Things that could be annoying in some way.

"I'm learning cane travel," I responded, "and I'll be out there on the street in Louisiana, walking with my instructor, and someone will walk up to me and take my arm and want to help me across the street. And I know they do that because they're being kind, but I don't need them to take my arm and help me walk across the street. It would be nicer if they would ask if I needed assistance or help. Most of us really want to do it on our own; it's kind of like going on a treasure hunt for me. It's a game—can I do it on my own?"

—⁂—

The last question Mr. Koppel asked me was something I had hinted at during the course of our two interviews: Was there anything about being blind that I actually liked better than being sighted?

"Anything that I like better? I don't eat as much."

"Why?"

"Because I can't see the food. I can't see the food, so I'm not tempted . . ."

With that Mr. Koppel said that I had been "absolutely charming," and that he was "so delighted" that I came in and he thanked me very much."

This was the first time that I know of that *ABC Nightline* aired two programs on the same subject back to back. The shows were a big success, and we felt they brought favorable attention to the blind and visually impaired as well as to our goals.

Quite a bit of the second program was dedicated to the activities and purpose of the NFB. We were pleased to help spread the word to the many blind and visually impaired who are unaware of what's available for them through organizations such as the NFB to help them achieve their goals.

Shortly after the Nightline interviews, I returned to the LCB to complete my education

In mid-August we took a field trip to a horse stable, and I was really excited; I love horseback riding.

I mounted the horse with no problem, but when someone placed the bridle in my hands, I immediately panicked: *Oh, my God! I can't see!* I had never thought about being unable to see on this horse, until I was holding the reins. I was sure I was going to fall, but one of the attendants said, "You can do this!" And he was right!

We rode all over the countryside for about an hour—across a brook, up and down hills. During the entire trip, my horse never floundered, and a branch never brushed against me. I was so proud of myself and felt empowered: *I did not give up; I completed the ride.*

Back at school, all the students began preparations for passing final exams. My Kitchen class required two "finals": preparing a dinner for twelve people and then a four-course meal for thirty. My meal for twelve was simple, and I got through it in a flash. For the larger dinner, I decided to make Greek food, because it's my favorite, and I have quite a bit of experience preparing it. I chose my menu: Greek salad, moussaka (a lasagna-like layering of eggplant and meat covered with a cream sauce), pita bread, and baklava for dessert.

To pass the final, every dish had to be made from scratch. That meant I had to find a recipe for even the pita bread, and bake it. No sweat. However, when I got to the moussaka, as I took the pan with the cream sauce off the stove, I dropped it! Now this was moussaka for thirty-five people. We are not talking about some little pot. It splashed down in the stove, all over the floor, and sprayed the cabinets. It splattered everywhere. I stood there stunned, wooden spoon in hand, and began to cry. However, my compassionate instructor took off at once for the store to get what I needed to make another batch. I pulled myself together, finished preparing the menu, and passed the class with a well-praised meal.

I never did really excel at Braille, due to numb fingers, but I learned all of the class-one Braille, A to Z, numbers one to ten, and punctuation. Of course, my speed was only about eight words a minute, but that didn't concern me. I just wanted to graduate!

I'd been dreading Wood Shop, but I was able to weasel out of it. I used the time allotted for Wood Shop for Braille and computer time because those classes were more important to me.

The last class to pass was Mobility. I was terrified of what my final would be. Fortunately, Roland had mercy on me and gave me a very light task, which I passed. So after five and a half months I graduated from the Louisiana Center for the Blind. *Hallelujah!* As I look back over my time there, in spite of my foot-dragging, outspokenness, reluctance to adhere to proven methods, and my struggle to accept being blind, the tenacity and compassion of the instructors finally broke through. I left the school with self-confidence and the firm conviction that I could accomplish anything I set my mind to. I had changed from a dependent blind woman to an independent woman who happened to be blind!

It's normally bitter medicine that does one the most good. Many of the students seemed to love LCB. But I, for one, found it bitter medicine indeed. However, I don't think I would be the person I am today without the NFB, and especially Boot Camp at LCB. I highly recommend it, and the other fine NFB schools, to any person who is blind or is losing his or her vision.

Don drove down from Alabama for my graduation on October 15, 1999. Afterward, we packed my many accumulated possessions into boxes and headed back to our Huntsville home, on the road to a brand new chapter.

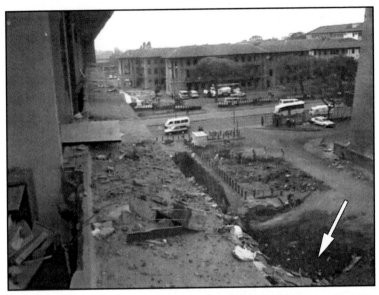

Behind the Nairobi embassy; arrow shows where the truck exploded[7]

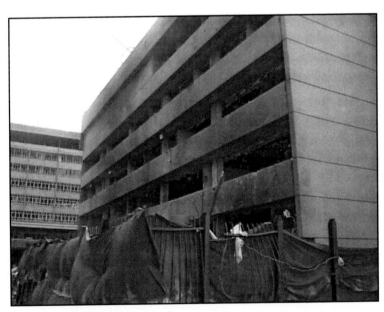

Back wall of the embassy showing blast burns. [7]
Ellen's office was near the center of this wall, partially below ground.

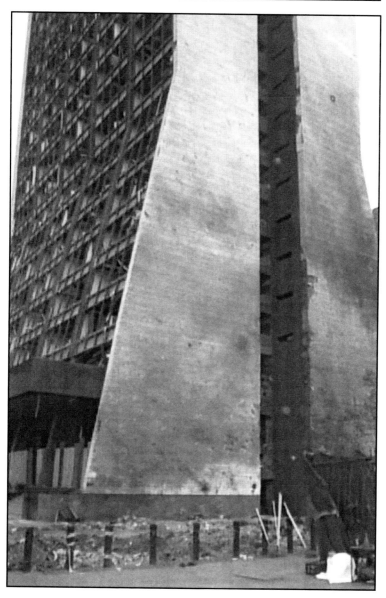

The nearby Kenya Commercial Bank building showing blast burns and shattered windows. U.S. Ambassador Bushnell was attending a meeting in a top floor office when the bomb detonated.[7]

CHAPTER 8

ORANGE JUICE
NEVER LOOKED
BETTER

EVEN THOUGH I struggled through LCB, I enjoyed a new sense of independence, and I wanted to continue living as normally as I could back in Huntsville. I still needed a certain amount of assistance, and Don had plenty to do without having to take me shopping or help me work out. So I hired Angie Slack as my assistant. She drove me wherever I needed to go, read to me, lifted weights with me, and generally helped me regain a sense of normalcy at home.

I knew I had to find an eye and ear doctor to continue my healing. Dr. Blair, my ear doctor at Walter Reed, recommended a colleague of hers in Birmingham, Alabama—Dr. Grayson Rodgers. I had no idea where to go for an eye specialist. I decided to ask our family dentist, Dr. James Pignatero, if he knew of anyone. (Only God knows why I thought a dentist would be able to recommend an eye specialist!) He recommended a local eye specialist, who recommended I go to Dr. Robert Phillips, a cornea specialist in Birmingham. I called these two doctors and set up appointments.

Dr. Rodgers examined my right ear and felt he might need to redo the eardrum replacement. I had exploratory surgery in November, and it was a complete success—no replacement was necessary.

In December, Dr. Phillips recommended I have a cornea transplant, but first he wanted me to be seen by the retina specialists: Drs. Robert Morris and Douglas Witherspoon. These two physicians not only specialize in eye trauma, they also developed specialized techniques that are utilized in only a few places around the world. They recommended that I undergo surgery at the end of the month with all three doctors, each focusing on his own specialty.

The surgeons started with my left eye. In ten hours of surgery, they repaired the retina, which contained quite a bit of scar tissue, and then did a cornea transplant.

Initially, I couldn't see anything with the repaired eye, which is normal. However, several days later I realized I was seeing double again, which meant my eye was working. When I tried to watch TV, all I could see was two big blurs separated vertically by a couple feet. It wasn't much, but it was progress. Once my vision returned to the best it was going to be, the doctors said they would operate on my eye muscles to correct the alignment. Dr. Phillips wanted to do a lens implant, which is the same basic procedure as cataract surgery, but there was too much damage to the cup that holds the lens behind the iris. However, he thought he might implant a lens in front of the iris at a later date. (The lenses were removed from both eyes during initial surgery in 1998, due to trauma-induced cataracts and the necessity to see inside the eye for repair to the retinas.)

When I returned to Birmingham for a checkup, the doctors were pleased with the results of the surgery. They said I had better than a 50/50 chance of recovering "useable" vision in my left eye. They also told me they would soon like to operate on my right eye, which had an even better chance of functioning again. Don and I harbored hopes that I would be able to read and watch TV again, even if only large print and big screen. At that point, we were happy to take whatever God saw fit to give us.

After many appointments and discussions, we decided to go ahead with the surgery to reattach the retina and replace the cornea in my right eye. We contacted *Nightline* to update them, and they sent a videographer to record the surgery and the end result.

I was very tense when the eye bandages were removed at my checkup following the surgery, and then so elated when I could actually "see" Dr. Morris, that I blurted out, "Hey, you're pretty good-looking!" He kindly smiled and then placed a can in front of me. I could actually read that it was Welch's Orange Juice. I don't think I have ever been quite so ecstatic at the sight of orange juice. That little can was proof I wasn't going to be blind!

A week or so later Don took me for another checkup. Drs. Witherspoon and Morris suggested I get fitted for glasses. That same day we went to an optometrist in Huntsville, and after they did a lot of lens swapping and flipping I was able to read a couple of characters on the 20/50 line of the near chart. Those letters are about three-sixteenths of an inch high, far better than I had been able to read any time since the bombing. I could only see one or two degrees horizontally, and I had to focus on each letter individually, but I really did have "useable" vision. They said to come back in a couple of days (No one-hour service for "Coke-bottle bottoms," I guess).

When my glasses were finally available, we made the trip to pick them up filled with apprehension. We had no idea what to expect. I took a deep breath and put on my new glasses. I could see even better than during the exam! My field of vision was still quite narrow, but I could read twelve-point type (about the size used in this book).

As we left the store, I saw green and red traffic lights for the first time in more than two years. Even though thrilled with all this improvement, I still thought it best for Don to drive us out to dinner to celebrate!

After dinner we went home and watched a movie. I could see the larger images, but it was still a bit difficult to follow the story when the camera panned back to encompass an entire scene. I got up and went into the kitchen for a snack. What a joy to read the labels on the cans and boxes in the pantry! I could even read the notes on the refrigerator! What was once a mundane grocery list had become for me as enthralling as a best-selling suspense thriller.

To our disappointment, however, my vision deteriorated by January, and I was relying more and more on my cane for "eyes." I had been asked to become a board member of the Alabama Institute for the Deaf and Blind (AID&B) and went there weekly for computer training. On one of those occasions, while using my cane to make my way down our driveway from our hilltop home to await a taxi, I heard someone urgently shout, "Ellen, stop!" Alarmed, I halted immediately, and then slowly backed up to wait on the front steps. Seems I was heading right off a six-foot drop beside my driveway, and discovered later that nobody had called my name! The warning surely came as a godsend.

Mid-May found me under the surgeon's knife once again. Apparently, the trauma of surgery in December reactivated scar tissue from the original injury, causing the retina in my right eye to detach again. Dr. Witherspoon relieved the tension on the retina and filled the eye with silicone oil to keep it in place. He told me my vision would be as good as it was before the detachment, but that I would have to get a new prescription for my glasses. It seems the oil bends light differently than the natural eye fluid does.

A couple days after the surgery the local chapter of the National Federation of the Blind (NFB) in Huntsville, Alabama, held a welcome-home dinner for me at the Hilton. I suggested we also make it a fundraiser so that Alabama could purchase NFB-Newsline for the blind in our state.

NFB-Newsline is a tool that allows a visually impaired person to call a toll-free number and have one of 250 newspapers or magazines read aloud. There is no charge to the user, and the person may read each newspaper, column to column and page to page, or choose individual sections. Hence, the visually impaired sports enthusiast can keep up with his favorite NBA team, a cook could read the recipes and try them, and a businessperson could stay informed on the latest financial news. Best of all, many local papers are available, so visually impaired individuals can keep up with what's going on in their own home towns. This opens up a whole new world for those who can't read conventional print, bringing them out of isolation and allowing them to become an active part of their communities.

The dinner proved to be wonderful. The mayor declared May fifteenth to be "Ellen Bomer Day" in Huntsville, Alabama. My doctors were present, family and friends, David and Rolph, our *Nightline* videographers, and many other supportive well-wishers totaling about 130 people. Best of all, we received more than a thousand dollars to begin funding NFB-Newsline for Alabama.

That seed money lit a fire in me, so several days later I contacted a friend of mine, Sybil Deschaines, who had connections within the state government, as well as lobbying experience. She and I went to Montgomery, the capital of Alabama, and met with a committee of lawmakers to ask that the state use excess monies from the fund that provides phone services for the hearing and speech impaired, to bring NFB-Newsline to Alabama. This precedent had already been set in other states, so we were simply asking them to follow suit. After nearly a year of discussion and debate, we were elated to learn that the state congress had passed the proposal—and continues to fund the service to this day.

Summer and fall passed uneventfully. I could see well enough to do most of what I needed to do and some of what I wanted to do. We were surprised to discover that I could read large-print playing cards, so we often got together with friends to play bridge. I also loved to bake and kept the pantry full of treats. Don loved it too—until he got on the scale.

In early December, my left eye rejected the transplanted cornea. The doctors weren't sure if trying again was wise, because the optic nerve was so badly damaged. And even with a new cornea, my vision in that eye would be limited at best.

A week or so later, we went back to Birmingham for yet another surgery on my right eye. The doctors had planned to remove the silicone oil and remove any scar tissue that may have formed on the retina, and they hoped to implant a permanent lens. The implant process is the same one done to those undergoing cataract surgeries, which is typically not a big deal. With me, however, they wanted to be sure that my eye had healed as much as it was going to before they proceeded. Otherwise, more scar tissue would likely develop and the risk of the body rejecting the transplant increased.

Unfortunately, when Dr. Witherspoon removed the oil from my eye, the retina again detached. Again, scar tissue was the culprit. To flatten the retina, he removed two tiny pieces (about 1 millimeter by .25 millimeter each) of the tension bands that were causing the problem, then replaced the oil and closed me up.

We hoped to try again in a few months, but they told me I'm "unique," and healing takes about two to four times longer for me than for a typical patient. Dr. Witherspoon informed us that the body eventually stops producing scar tissue, so we had reason to believe that the next operation would be the "one."

The year ended on that hope-filled note. Unfortunately, mountaintops lead to valleys, and I had yet another valley awaiting me in New York City: testifying at the trial of the terrorists who planned and executed the embassy bombings.

CHAPTER 9

THE TRIAL

BY MARCH OF 2000, my vision had deteriorated to mere shadows and shapes. For that reason, among others, I was looking forward to my upcoming surgery—the one we hoped would be the last on my right eye. This operation would be a second attempt at a lens implant, and along with that, replacement of the silicone oil with a more natural fluid. As I mentioned before, the lens implant is a common procedure performed in cataract surgery. In that case, the natural lens is removed from behind the iris, leaving a "capsule" in which a plastic lens is placed. In my case, however, there was no capsule, nor was there a functioning iris. They were planning to sew the lens in place. We weren't sure what they were going to sew the lens onto, but we had complete faith in Dr. Witherspoon and his team.

The doctor told me I would notice instant significant improvement in vision. Then the eye would require about three months to recover from the trauma of surgery and become stable. Potentially, I could end up with 20/50 vision (corrected and good enough to possibly drive!) in my right eye.

The day of the surgery, Dr. Witherspoon expressed his concern about finding a suitable place to attach the lens implant. This particular implant has two small legs that twist away from the center, much like cloud bands from a hurricane. Because my iris had scar tissue from one o'clock to three o'clock, so to speak, and that was the area where he needed to attach the lens, he wasn't quite sure what he was going to do. (He could not attach it to scar tissue.) He said to me, "Ellen, please pray. That's all we can do. God is going to have to make a space."

Don told me later that Dr. Witherspoon had approached him after the surgery, wearing a gigantic smile. He had found a spot no more than three hair-widths wide—just what he needed—in exactly the right place! The surgery was a success!

After he finished repairing my eye, the doctor returned to the operating room to remove seven pieces of glass from my forehead—all but one were about 3/16 by 1/8 of an inch in size. To this accomplished micro surgeon, these slivers of glass looked like boulders!

In the spring of 2000, the trial of Mohamed Rashed Daoud Al-'Owhali, Khalfan Khamis, Mohamed Sadeek Odeh, and Wadih El Hage filled seventy-six days and nearly nine thousand pages of transcript. These four men shared responsibility for carrying out Osama bin Laden's orders to bomb the two United States embassies—one in Kenya and one in Tanzania. These combined actions resulted in the deaths of approximately 224 persons, and injuring more than 5,000.

I had received an invitation from the U.S. Attorney General's office to attend the trial simply as an observer for a week, and even though I dreaded the experience, I thought it might help bring closure.

My sister-in-law, Trish, accompanied me to New York City, where we stayed at the Marriott Twin Towers, unaware of the foreshadowing, of course, that in a short time our hotel's namesakes would be destroyed and more lives lost at the instigation of Osama bin Laden.

Each day federal agents transported us to the courthouse, through metal detectors, and into the courtroom.

We sat hour after hour, listening to the closing arguments of both sides. The prosecutor began his summary with these words:[3]

> What does the evidence show that the defendant Wadih El Hage did in connection with this conspiracy? Now, in his opening statement, counsel for El Hage, on behalf of El Hage, said to you that Mr. El Hage was a mediator and that he was somebody who shared in the tragedy of the embassy bombings. Ladies and gentlemen, I submit to you that the evidence shows that Wadih El Hage was a facilitator, somebody who performed key logistical acts on behalf of the Al-Qaeda conspiracy and somebody who obstructed the investigation into Al-Qaeda within a year of the bombing and within weeks after the bombing.
>
> What the evidence shows, ladies and gentlemen, is that, like many people in Al-Qaeda, Wadih El Hage has a family and that Wadih El Hage conducts business transactions. But like other people in Al-Qaeda, the evidence shows

that Wadih El Hage led a double life, a secret criminal life on behalf of Al-Qaeda, and that he performed logistical services for Al-Qaeda to make sure that others in Al-Qaeda could carry out their deadly acts.

The evidence shows that as far back as 1992 and 1993 Wadih El Hage was in charge of the Al-Qaeda payroll in Khartoum, Sudan, when Al-Qaeda was headquartered in that country. It showed that Wadih El Hage made efforts to transport Stinger Missiles from Pakistan to Sudan in 1993, the same year that Al-Qaeda was targeting the American peace-keeping mission in Somalia, and the evidence shows that Wadih El Hage arranged for the transport of five Al-Qaeda people from Khartoum down to Nairobi, also during the time that Al-Qaeda was targeting the American presence in Somalia.

What else does the evidence show? The evidence shows that Wadih El Hage served as Osama bin Laden's personal assistant, the gatekeeper to the man that was the head of this secret conspiracy. The evidence also shows that in 1994 Wadih El Hage moved from Khartoum, Sudan down to Nairobi, Kenya to become a leader of the East African cell of Al-Qaeda.

And the evidence shows that when he got down to Nairobi, he maintained a close operational working relationship with the East African cell—and, ladies and gentlemen, this is the same cell that would carry out the bombings of the embassies in Nairobi and Dar es Salaam; that Wadih El Hage arranged for the facilitation and delivery of false travel documents of other Al-Qaeda members; that he communicated in code and passed on messages to others in Al-Qaeda; that he maintained a close working relationship with others in the East African cell, such as the defendant, Mohamed Odeh.

And in 1997 you heard evidence that Wadih El Hage went twice to visit Osama bin Laden and his commander, Abu Hafs, here in Afghanistan. And when he returned from that first trip in February of 1997, Wadih El Hage brought back with him a new policy, a policy to militarize, to militarize the cell that in sixteen or eighteen months thereafter would carry out the bombings in East Africa.

And then you heard that El Hage went back to see Bin Laden in August of 1997, a year after Bin Laden had publicly declared war against the United States, six months after he gave the interview with CNN where he said he would send dead Americans home. And when El Hage returned, he was met by American officials and he testified before a grand jury in this courthouse, when the American government was conducting an investigation of Al-Qaeda to try to learn about what Al-Qaeda was doing in its war against America, to try to stop Al-Qaeda from carrying out its deadly mission.

And it was at that moment that Wadih El Hage was faced with a choice: He could honor his oath, he could tell the truth, he could help the United States against Al-Qaeda, or he could side with Al-Qaeda and Bin Laden. And the evidence overwhelmingly establishes that what Wadih El Hage did was he sided with Jihad, he sided with Al-Qaeda. The American citizen chose Bin Laden over America. And he would do it again, because the evidence shows that in 1998, merely weeks after our embassies were bombed, Wadih El Hage testified again before the grand jury and again he took an oath and again he chose Al-Qaeda over the United States. And he lied about key members of Al-Qaeda, and one of the people that he lied about was the defendant, Mohamed Odeh, which is where we turn next.

What does the evidence show about Mohamed Odeh? The evidence shows, ladies and gentlemen, that Mohamed Odeh was a sworn member of Al-Qaeda, that he was a sworn member of Al-Qaeda since 1992; that he maintained his status as a sworn and paid member of Al-Qaeda through the various fatwahs and declarations of Jihad issued by Osama bin Laden; that he maintained his status as a sworn and paid member of Al-Qaeda through August 7th, 1998. Mohamed Odeh received extensive training in Afghanistan in firearms, in explosives such as TNT, and he received advance explosive training at Al-Qaeda's camps.

The evidence also shows, ladies and gentlemen, that Mohamed Odeh trained ideologically similar groups in Somalia, once again at the same time while Al-Qaeda was targeting the American presence in Somalia.

The evidence also shows that Mohamed Sadeek Odeh was given a business, a fishing business, by the military commander of Al-Qaeda, a man by the name of Abu Hafs, and that Mohamed Odeh remained an active member of the East African cell of Al-Qaeda, maintaining contact and working with Wadih El Hage and others. And some of the others that he worked with carried out the bombings and he carried them out with them.

In particular, ladies and gentlemen, the evidence shows that Mohamed Odeh attended several meetings in the spring and the summer of 1998, with the very same people who carried out the bombing, and what you will see and what the evidence shows is that Mohamed Odeh's role was as the technical advisor to those who carried out the bombing in Nairobi.

The evidence also shows that Mohamed Odeh traveled to Nairobi in the days before the bombing. He checked into a hotel using a fake name, supported by a fake passport; that he attended meetings where he knew that Al-Qaeda was expecting American retaliation for something that Al-Qaeda was about to do; and that he fled Nairobi the night before the bombing, using that fake passport, on his way to Afghanistan, the headquarters of Al-Qaeda and the home of Osama bin Laden, and that he was caught on the morning of August 7th in Pakistan.

Now, the evidence shows that Mohamed al-'Owhali had a very different role in this case. Mohamed al-'Owhali was to carry out the attack. He was the person who was supposed to execute the bombing in Nairobi, and you know from the evidence that he was supposed to die in the bombing.

Now, what the evidence shows is that Mohamed al-'Owhali also received training at Al-Qaeda camps in Afghanistan. He learned about explosives, he learned about weapons, but he also learned about hijackings, he learned about kidnappings, and he was proficient enough at this training to earn an audience with Osama bin Laden. And it was during one of his meetings with Osama bin Laden that Mohamed al-'Owhali asked for a mission, a mission that you know he got and that you know he carried out, to the detriment of 213 people.

Now, Mohamed al-'Owhali, he, too, gets a fake passport and the evidence shows that he goes to Yemen in May of 1998 and then he goes back to Afghanistan, where he gets the details of where it is that the operation is supposed to be carried out. He made a video that was supposed to take credit for his martyrdom operation, a video that Al-Qaeda was going to show to celebrate its attack against the embassy in Nairobi. And then he got to Nairobi in the early days of August and he met with the other people that he was going to work with to carry out the bombing.

He did some last-minute surveillance of the embassy. He reviewed some photos and some sketches of the embassy. He learned all about the plan in Dar es Salaam, and then he was given his instructions. And what you know is he carried out his instructions.

On the morning of the bombing, in that back parking lot of the embassy, Mohamed al-'Owhali got out of the truck, he threw his flash grenades in an effort to get that truck as close to the target as possible—the American Embassy in Nairobi, Kenya.

Only the plan called for him to die, and he ran. And when he ran, and realizing he had no travel documents and that he had no money, he reached out to Al-Qaeda. He called Yemen, and Mohamed al-'Owhali and Al-Qaeda worked together to rescue al-'Owhali before he was apprehended in Nairobi, Kenya.

What does the evidence show about Khalfan Khamis Mohamed? The evidence shows that he, too, obtained the requisite training in Afghanistan and that he, too, went to Somalia to train others, but that in March of 1998 Khalfan Khamis Mohamed was approached about doing a Jihad job, a job he readily accepted, and that it was Khalfan Khamis Mohamed that purchased the utility vehicle, that white Suzuki that was used to transport the component of the bomb, the TNT, the gas cylinders, the detonators.

And you learned that Khalfan Khamis Mohamed rented that place, that house at 213 Ilala that functioned as the bomb factory where Khalfan Khamis Mohamed and the others ground the TNT and put together the bomb and loaded the bomb on the bomb truck so that it could be delivered to the American Embassy in Dar es Salaam. And you know that Khalfan Khamis Mohamed went with that bomb truck and he prayed that the bomb would go off, and he was happy when it did. And Khalfan Khamis Mohamed cleaned up the house in an effort to erase the trail that would connect him and his cohorts in the bombing and he fled to South Africa.

Now, ladies and gentlemen, that was just a brief summary of what the evidence shows that these four defendants did, what it is that they did that makes them guilty of the charges that have been brought against them in this indictment.[3]

—◦◦◦—

Hearing the facts laid out in such a cut-and-dried manner, and to hear how cold, calculating, and focused these men had been—brought tears to our eyes and pain once again to our hearts.

At the same time as the trial, I was also interviewed by a reporter from the Associated Press. After the week was up, my sister-in-law and I returned to our respective homes in Alabama and Texas, and a few days later we both read the AP story which had been picked up by newspapers all over the world.[4]

—◦◦◦—

The article told how I sat in a federal courtroom, blinded by terrorism, listening for justice. With my cane I sat a few feet from the four men responsible for carrying out bin Laden's orders to destroy the American Embassy in Nairobi, as it detailed the number who were injured and died.

"It's like listening to an audio book,"' I told them, describing the sounds of the four-month old trial as it approached its conclusion with closing arguments.

I had come to hear the defendants explain themselves and take responsibility for their actions, intent upon hearing their testimony. And my desire was not granted.

"I wanted to hear their voices because I can't see them. I was so disappointed they didn't testify," I admitted.

Dramatically, the article pointed out that I now waited to hear the voice of the jury deal its hand.

"I am anxious to hear that justice is done. That is the word I want to hear: guilty. It will never be enough because of what they have taken from all of us," I told them. "They have invaded our lives and stolen from us things we can never, ever replace."

The article continued to speak of my faithful attendance and intent listening as I, a Pennsylvania native, at age fifty-four, sat among the other survivors and relatives of victims. It then followed through with my own story, and what had happened to me as a result of the terrorists' attack on our lives.

Toward the conclusion of the article, I asked of the bombings, "What purpose did this serve? I want to know why."

I related how I had gotten some relief from listening to testimony, and expected the two truck drivers to get the death penalty, anticipating I would take the stand once the penalty phase began for the convicted men.

Not angry, I told them, "I'm really in a quandary to understand why. I don't want revenge. I want accountability. I want them to step up and say, 'We did this.' They should suffer the consequences of their actions quickly."

"I still have that fire inside of me," I said. "They won't beat us. They won't ever defeat us."

Shortly after my return home, I developed a pneumococcus infection in my eye. More doctor visits. More eye drops. It barely even fazed me anymore.

In early June, I returned to New York City to testify in the sentencing of the perpetrators. My cousin Constantina Crusade accompanied me this time, and we stayed in a different hotel farther away from the courthouse, which seemed to be more closely guarded.

This time it was extremely difficult to sit in the courtroom and listen to the testimony of my co-workers and the surviving dependents of employees who died. It was my first time listening to their stories. And it was heartbreaking. My resolve was strengthened to be a good witness.

In addition to the emotional trauma, I also struggled physically. My newly acquired vision was starting to deteriorate, and I needed my long white cane again. I was still fighting the invasive infection. This meant I had to put drops in my eye every hour. The drops required refrigeration, so I carried a thermos everywhere.

On the day I was to testify, while waiting for transport to the courthouse in the hotel lobby, the doctor who attended me in Landstuhl Army Medical Center in Germany approached me. "Mrs. Bomer," he exclaimed, "I would never have recognized you if I hadn't recalled your name. You look so much better than when I saw you last!" I thanked him, and my day was off to a positive start.

Later on, as I waited to testify in a room near the courtroom, I felt on edge with both trepidation and hope. I had never been a witness in a trial before, and I knew my statement had the potential to affect the outcome of the proceedings. I was determined to present a strong and compelling testimony regarding the pain and suffering experienced by survivors of the bombing.

I was sworn in and the prosecutor began his questioning. I described what happened to me and how it affected my life and my family. Several times, I tearfully testified that I was only an employee of the U.S. government doing my job, and in no way was I a threat to Al-Qaeda, or anybody. I avowed that I would never be defeated by this dreadful bombing, and that Osama bin Laden did not "win." I was blind, yes, but I was not beaten!

I truly believe, to move on in life, "winners" decide they are "survivors" and take on the tough responsibilities which empower them, instead of continuing to play the powerless victim role. My focus on God enabled me to have the courage to do just that!

After testifying, I left the courtroom, but my cousin stayed. She told me later that the defense attorney rose and declared "no more victim impact testimony was necessary." He told the judge, "Mrs. Bomer's testimony would make a stone weep."

The judge overruled the DA's objection, and I returned to the courtroom to hear more testimonies; more stories of loss, pain, and death.

When the guilty verdict was read, it felt as if the whole courtroom exhaled. We believed the men would be convicted, but we weren't jumping to conclusions just yet.

A few months later, Don and I received word of the sentences: life in prison without parole. According to reports, some of the jurors expressed concerns that executing the men might elevate them to "martyr" status within Islam, thereby making heroes of them. The four men are currently incarcerated at the United States Penitentiary Administrative Maximum Facility (ADX) in Florence, Colorado. It is our understanding that they will spend their time in solitary confinement—twenty-three hours a day, every day for the rest of their lives. Perhaps that is a more fitting punishment for their crimes.

CHAPTER 10

FROM THE ASHES

DON AND I were eating dinner together one night, and he said, "Look at me."

I turned to face him.

"Something's not right," he said. He had noticed a small white spot near the center of my cornea. The pneumococcus infection of a few weeks earlier ate a pit in my cornea called a corneal ulcer. It took about a month to kill the infecting bacteria, and the damage it caused rendered my corneal graft completely useless. The graft had been cloudy, and we knew it would probably need to be replaced, but this ulcer guaranteed it. So, in mid July, I found myself once again on the operating table.

After nearly six hours of surgery, I had a new cornea. The eye doctors informed Don that there were no signs of scarring, retinal detachment, or internal infection. I was also given another "oil change," because my eye was still not producing the fluid needed to increase internal pressure, keep the retina in place, and retain the shape of my eyeball.

Oddly enough, medications exist to help lower eye pressure, such as those used by people with glaucoma, but there's nothing available to raise pressure.

Although this procedure was seemingly successful, my vision did not return after post-operative healing. Rather, it continued to very slowly deteriorate towards blackness over the next couple of months.

One Tuesday in mid-August Don came home from work terribly sick with a bad summer cold. We ate dinner and watched TV for a while. I'd had a headache most of the afternoon, so I took a Motrin, and then fell asleep for a half hour or so.

When I woke up, I sat up and said, "I hav a frsmiple yuop."

Don looked at me like I'd grown a second nose during my nap, and said, "What?"

I repeated what I believed was a perfectly clear sentence: "I hav a blwract zfrg."

After my third attempt at communicating, Don leaped into action. He said, "We're going to the hospital—now!" Fortunately, he recognized the signs of a stroke. He handed me a couple of aspirins (appropriate "first response" to treat a stroke or heart attack victim), led me to the car, and off we went.

Still minutes from the emergency room, I told Don my right arm and the right side of my mouth were numb. With that announcement, Don moved from simply breaking the speed limit to breaking the sound barrier.

By the time we arrived at the hospital, I no longer had any symptoms. Regardless, the nurse wheeled me down the hall for a CT scan. (I will always have too much metal in my body to get an MRI.)

The following morning brought more tests: an EEG, an EKG, and who knows how many more three-letter procedures. The results showed no damage or continuing symptoms. The doctors weren't positive of the diagnosis, but it's likely I experienced a TIA, a Transient Ischemic Attack, essentially a mini-stroke . . . and another three letters!

I went home that afternoon, with instructions to take one coated 350-milligram aspirin every day for the rest of my life. Compared to my other hospital experiences, this one was a piece of cake!

The next day, with Don even sicker with viral symptoms he was now generously sharing with me, our son Michael's partner, Amy, gave birth to our first granddaughter: Alexandra (Allie) Rain Cormier. Because of our colds, we could not see her until later in the week, and then had to wear masks.

She was undoubtedly the most beautiful baby in the nursery, but regrettably, I had lost all my restored vision, and had to content myself with gently touching her face, fingers, and toes. She felt so warm and soft, and I couldn't help but thank God for this precious little one He had brought into our lives.

The week after Allie was born, I went to our family doctor for a blood draw. Apparently in the craziness of dealing with my stroke symptoms, the hospital hadn't run appropriate tests on my blood.

A few days later, the nurse called to say our doctor wanted to see me. My blood showed positive for ANA, a possible indicator of lupus.

Don was with me when the doctor informed us it probably wasn't lupus, but that several medications, including some I took, could cause a positive ANA reading. However, another symptom of lupus is frequent, painless mouth ulcers, or canker sores. I definitely had frequent canker sores, but they weren't painless. The doctor said he wanted to hold off on treatment for the time being, and just wait and see if any further symptoms manifested.

Nine days after Allie's birth, my friend Nancy Cooper and I were out shopping when my cell phone rang. The caller identified herself as a social worker from the Department of Human Resources. "I've just returned from a visit to your son's apartment," she said. "Because I found illegal drugs there, I was obligated remove the child from the home. Are you willing to take custody of her? If not, we'll have to place her in foster care."

I had been pretty focused on finding my next perfect pair of shoes, so I was still trying to process the words "social worker" and "Department of Human Resources." My brain had not begun to wrap itself around "custody" and "foster care"—and she wanted an answer to her question.

"Say that again, please?"

She repeated her explanation and request.

I still did not completely comprehend all of the implications of what she was asking, nonetheless, the woman was talking about my grandchild. I didn't even have to think twice. "Of course, we'll take her. When do you want to bring her over?"

"Now."

"Now?!"

"Yes."

Well, she got right to the point. I had to give her that.

"I'll be home in thirty minutes," I told her.

As Nancy drove me home, my mind was racing faster than her car engine. I had just enough time to put down my packages and gulp down a glass of iced tea before the doorbell rang.

Allie arrived with a few diapers, some formula, and the layette I had bought for her before she was born. We had set up a portable crib a few days earlier for Allie's anticipated visits, not knowing she would be using it this soon!

The social worker placed Allie in my arms, told me she'd be in touch, and walked out the door.

Apprehension and uncertainty sloshed around with the iced tea in my stomach. *God, is this why you spared my life? Maybe this is what I'm supposed to do—not rock anonymous babies in the hospital, but care for my own granddaughter. But, God, my "baby" is thirty-four years old. It's been a long time! And, by the way God, I'm blind, remember? How will I take care of a baby?*

Providentially, my mother was visiting that week, and she came to my rescue: putting clothes in drawers, preparing formula, stacking diapers, and generally tending the baby for the first few days. It was all I could do to just hold Allie. I was so afraid I'd drop her!

Finally, the baby needed a bath and my mother wasn't physically up to that task. I remembered my training in Louisiana: *If I can find my way through a strange town, over railroad tracks, through swarms of stinging ants in the rain—I can give this child a bath!*

Both Allie and I survived her first bath—and the many that followed. Our next crisis came when she was about five months old: How would I feed her with a spoon? It's one thing to give a bottle to a tiny infant who's lying still in my arms. It's quite another to put a spoon into the mouth of a squirming, independent baby who'd rather be down on the floor scooting around.

I consulted with a friend at the Alabama Institute for the Deaf and Blind and received excellent advice. He told me to hold Allie on my lap with her back against my chest. I could gently hold her lower jaw with one hand, and feed her with the other.

With an old-fashioned cloth diaper clothes-pinned around her neck (we needed something bigger than a standard bib!), Allie sat on my lap just as the teacher had suggested. Her mouth was like a little bird's—always open! And if the food didn't find its target fast enough, she would turn her head to find the spoon.

By the end of that first lap-meal, more strained peaches went into Allie's mouth than onto her bib, I'm proud to say. We both left the table happy: Allie with a full tummy, and me with added confidence that I really could care for my granddaughter, even if I could not see her.

When Allie began to crawl, we faced another challenge. This one had a simple solution, however. Some people put bells on their cats; we put bells on Allie's shoes. Day after day, she and I crawled around the house, exploring together. It was a new experience for both of us, and lifted any depression. I was preoccupied with taking care of this precious gift from God!

Thanksgiving of 2001 brought many reasons for gratitude.

Though I had lost vision in my left eye, Dr. Witherspoon remained pleased with the progress of healing.

One more corneal graft on my right eye, completed only the week before, seemed to be a success. The surgeons found no surprises, and they expected me to regain at least some sight in that eye.

Best of all, we had Allie. Not only was she growing and thriving, her presence had brought new purpose and meaning to my days. Anyone who's raised a child may look back and wish different decisions or actions had been taken on certain occasions. We all have some regrets, be they big or small, when it comes to our children. Perhaps raising Allie would be an opportunity for us to parent differently, hopefully better. The embassy bombing changed our lives in many obvious ways, but it had also made us wiser, stronger, and more focused. We hoped Allie would benefit from our experiences. Perhaps we would receive, in the words of the ancient prophet, Isaiah, "beauty for ashes" after all.

CHAPTER 11

WHEN POSITIVE IS
NEGATIVE

I LOWERED THE car window just a crack and inhaled deeply. There's nothing quite like the smell of spring—and spring in the mountains of Tennessee is even better.

My dear friend Nancy Cooper described the passing scenery as she, Allie, and I journeyed through Knoxville to Helen, Georgia, for a week of refreshing relaxation.

On our first day after arriving, we visited the Cabbage Patch Hospital, where the dolls are made and sold. Our tour began where the dolls are "born." The room is designed to look like an actual cabbage patch, and each cabbage holds a doll. We then proceeded upstairs to the nursery, where it sounds as though the dolls are breathing gently as they sleep. In her stroller, Allie responded to this, making small sounds, as if she were communicating with other babies.

We "adopted" one of the dolls, Lucy Jeannette. I planned to put the doll away until Allie graduated from kindergarten. Being a grandma is so much fun!

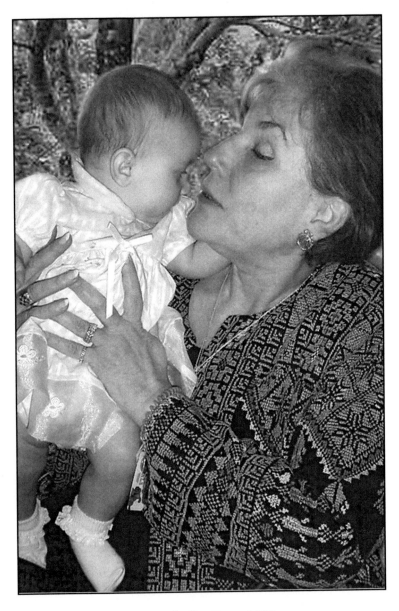

Ellen and Allie, Easter 2002.

We spent the rest of the week exploring downtown shops and sampling delicious German cuisine at various restaurants.

Nancy and I are both weavers and knitters and took tactile delight in a specialty yarn shop. I purchased some of the sumptuous fibers for a knitting project, because I believed that I would eventually see well enough to do it again.

The week passed quickly and enjoyably. The only downside to the entire trip was a constant ache in my back. Probably from carrying Allie, so I didn't pay much attention to it.

The pain persisted upon our return, however, so a couple of months later I had it checked out. The doctor examined my back and my lungs and told me again that maybe I had lupus. It can be difficult to diagnose, so he wasn't sure.

I did not get any better, so I went back to see him in June. After a chest X-ray, he told me to check into the hospital. He needed to do a laparoscopy to look at my lungs.

Don admitted me into the hospital. Later that evening they took me to the operating room for the procedure. The last thing I heard was a nurse saying, "Pressure's forty over twenty."

I was dying.

The next thing I recall was waking up, but I wasn't really awake. I'm in this very bright room again and see people everywhere. And I'm thinking to myself, *Okay, John, I'm here.* And his reply was, *No, your birthday's coming. You've got to go back for your birthday.* And I remember thinking, *Oh, August first. Okay, they're going to have a party for me.* And John concurred with, *Yes, you have to go back.* That was the last thing I remembered.

I woke up four days later in intensive care. The doctor informed me I had been on a respirator the entire time, and that they'd not been able to do the laparoscopy. The medical staff did not know what was wrong with me. They told me that a priest had administered last rites. They really expected me to die.

I remained hospitalized for three weeks and was finally diagnosed with Acute Respiratory Distress Syndrome (ARDS).

By the time I was discharged, I was so weak I could barely walk. Don administered intravenous antibiotics twice a day, and a nurse came by three or four times a week to check the arterial IV I had to wear. After a week of these antibiotic drips I started to get better. Once again, God spared my life.

In mid July, I started running a low-grade fever in the evenings, and I seemed to be tired all the time.

After a week, I went back to the doctor. He did another chest X-ray, told me I had pneumonia, and sent me back to the hospital for a lung biopsy. After the procedure the surgeon told us my lungs looked more like liver tissue than lung tissue. Following the biopsy, I stayed in the hospital, where I received massive doses of antibiotics. The days of waiting for test results seem to drag by as slowly as a bad sermon.

Finally, another week later when Don was present, Dr. Leroy Harris, a communicable disease specialist, entered my room in the morning and, standing at the foot of my bed, informed us that I had Pneumocystis Carinii Pneumonia (PCP) and Cytomegalovirus Pneumonia (CMV)—brought on by an African strain of a blood-borne disease living in my body for the last four years. Did this come from lying for hours in blood and bodily fluids before being rescued? Did it come from my rescuers? Or even the blood-drenched hospitals I was first taken to? Only God knows for certain.

In the middle of recovering from this latest medical nightmare, Don and I were granted total and permanent parental custody of Allie. Though the task seemed daunting, the only reassurance I ever needed was when Allie snuggled into me as I gave her bottle. Her small movements and sighs of contentment communicated loud and clear: "Everything's going to be all right."

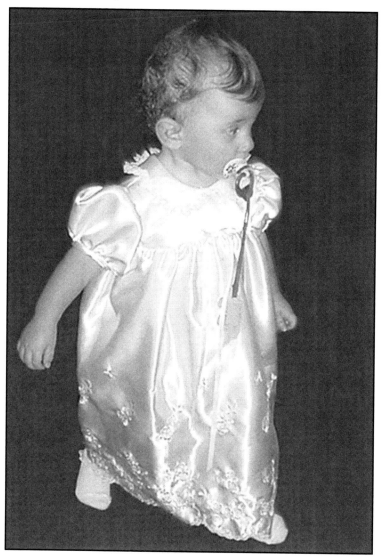

Allie on her baptism day, 2002

CHAPTER 12

A NEW OUTLOOK

IN SEPTEMBER OF 2003, I was honored to receive the Thomas Jefferson Star Award for Foreign Service. This Award is the highest presidential award a civilian Foreign Service employee can receive. Time had mellowed the drama we experienced before in Washington, D.C., and we had the privilege of hearing Secretary of State Colin Powell speak and meeting him personally following the ceremony. I appreciated being recognized for my service and for the injuries and disabilities that resulted from my time in Nairobi.

By late 2003, traffic on our street in Huntsville had become quite heavy, and we were robbed in our own driveway. Not feeling safe there anymore, I pressed Don to retire from COLSA Corporation, the same defense contractor he worked for in Saudi Arabia, and move to our little ranch in Wimberley, Texas. I don't think he was quite ready to retire, but he eventually agreed. And in March of 2004, we packed up our worldly goods and put down new roots in the Lone Star state.

A couple months after we settled in, Don had to go to Baltimore for a conference. Since we didn't really know anyone in Wimberley, I placed an ad in the local newspaper for someone who could work twenty to thirty hours a week, basically being my eyes.

A young woman named Teresa Cable answered the ad, and she's been both my assistant and my dear friend ever since.

By the end of that first summer, we were ready to find a church. We knew we were going to stay in Wimberley, so we wanted to establish ourselves, especially Allie, in the community. Initially, we did not experience much success in our search until we saw an ad for daycare and preschool at St. Stephen's Episcopal Church. Because we live out in the country, I believed it would be beneficial for Allie to go to daycare a couple mornings a week, be around other children, and develop friendships. So she was enrolled, and Don drove her to the church two days a week.

Allie loved her time with the kids at the daycare, and a month or so later, I told Don, "We should check out this church. Everybody seems so friendly and loving."

Don agreed, and it wasn't long before we began attending regularly. About a year later we formally joined the church.

I'm a gregarious person; I enjoy being around people. Just attending church on Sundays didn't quite fulfill my need for social interaction. When I discovered that the church sponsored a women's Bible study, I phoned the leader, Connie Maverick, and asked about joining the group.

"Of course!" she replied. "We'd be happy to have you."

She gave me the details of the upcoming meeting, and I coerced Teresa into going with me. Neither one of us had much knowledge of the Bible, so we were a little unsure of fitting in with this group.

We needn't have worried. The women accepted us warmly and made us feel right at home.

Teresa and I attended the study faithfully for the next two years, enjoying the camaraderie and soaking up more and more knowledge and wisdom from the Bible.

Toward the end of 2006, Connie approached me and asked me to lead the study.

"You're joking, right?"

"No, Ellen. I've thought about it, prayed about it, and I really think you're the person to take over."

I did not feel like I knew enough about the Bible yet to lead, but I knew that with Connie's confidence and God's help, I'd muddle through somehow. Of course, never one to be content with "muddling," I started attending a class called Education for Ministry, offered by St. Stephen's every Tuesday afternoon. The curriculum spans four years, and when students complete the course they have a good solid grounding in God's Word. It's been exciting to dig into the content and history of the Bible, and I know it's made me a better leader, and a better person!

Along with the Bible study and the Education for Ministry class, I also sang in the choir for a year or so. I hesitated a bit at first because I knew I wouldn't be able to see the music. But the director, Ann Jones, kindly assured me that we could work around it. Sure enough, we did. I went to rehearsals on Wednesday nights and recorded the pieces we'd be singing the following Sunday. I played the recording over and over, studying, listening, and singing along. Then on Sunday morning I was as prepared as any other choir member. Unfortunately, I had to drop choir

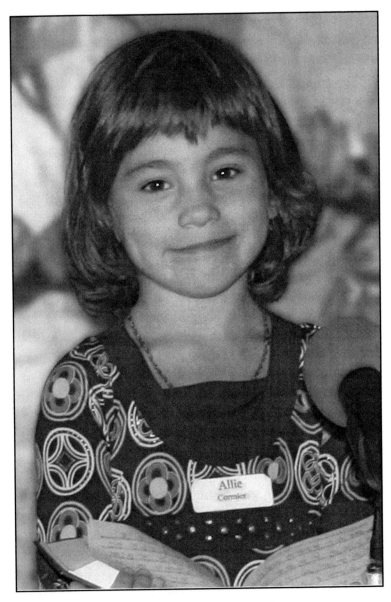

Allie singing in choir, 2008[8]

as Don was now running the church sound system and recording the service each week. This left Allie unattended and that's not what church should be, so I opted to sit with her during the service.

Allie followed in my footsteps and sang in the St. Stephens Children's Choir for a while. The children perform several times a year and it's such a joy to hear their young voices singing praises to God.

Now, as a nine-year-old, she takes time to talk to many of the older people in the church as well as the younger children. She shakes their hands, asks if they can be friends, and flashes her sweet smile—usually receiving one in return! What amazes me most is how much she's like her Uncle John. He, too, throughout his short life, would often stop to talk with elderly neighbors or other adults who did not often socialize. He would try to bring a smile from a warm handshake wherever he went. We miss him and feel blessed to have reminders of him in Allie.

People often ask me how I became blind, and when I tell them my story, their next question goes something like, "Well, what do you think of Osama bin Laden now? What would you say to him if you met him on the street?" I don't spend much time thinking about bin Laden, but when I do it's a bit abstract. After all, I don't know him personally—although I met a few of his countless sisters, aunts, and uncles when we lived in Jeddah. My experience with his family was nothing but positive and I found them to be kind and gracious people.

I believe in my heart that many, if not most, of Osama's family do not agree with his jihad. After all, black sheep are born into the best of flocks!

I know Osama bin Laden will have to answer for his actions someday, if not here on earth, then certainly before God. And I know that whatever retribution bin Laden deserves is something I am helpless to accomplish myself. I can only bear witness.

Do I hate him? No. Harboring hatred, bitterness, and resentment is destructive energy to one's self and lifestyle. And frankly, I'd much rather focus my attention and efforts on the good things in my story—my family, my church, and my friends.

Life is good, and my days center on caring for Allie. Most of the time I don't worry about being blind. I'm able to do everything I need to with Allie. Of course, I would like to read to her, or pick out her clothes, or even see her face. I have a mental picture of what she looks like—I'm told she looks just like her father, my son Michael—but I don't know when or if I'll be able to compare my image with the living, breathing reality of Allie on earth.

None of us knows what the future holds. And if I've learned anything, it's that our sense of control over our futures, our destinies, is an illusion. We play the hand we're dealt and leave the rest up to God. As for me, I continue to hope for vision, even as I live and enjoy each day God gives me.

CHAPTER 13

IN THEIR OWN WORDS

MANY PROFESSIONALS, FAMILY members, and friends have walked the steps of this journey with me, and this chapter is an opportunity for a few of them to share their thoughts and perspectives on the events you've just read about. I feel privileged to include their words alongside mine.

Dr. Douglas Witherspoon, M.D.

My associates and I specialize in dealing with eye trauma. We're not necessarily household names, but we've broken ground in the medical community in regard to developing new procedures for operating on eyes that have been simultaneously injured in the front and the back.

By the time I met Don and Ellen Bomer in November of 1999—some fourteen months after she had sustained her injuries—she had already undergone nine reconstructive eye surgeries, all attempts to restore her vision. Unfortunately, all she could see at the time was a bit of light.

In December of that year, we performed a "temporary keratoprosthesis vitrectomy" on her left eye (then the right eye in May 2000), a procedure that my colleagues and I spent about fifteen years developing. Briefly, here's how it works. When the retina is badly damaged, it's necessary to operate by looking through the cornea of the eye using a high-powered microscope, and then inserting instruments into the back of the eye, lighting it up from the inside using a fiber-optic illuminator. In this way we can repair damage, remove scar tissue, and do any other necessary procedures.

Ellen's cornea, however, was completely cloudy as a result of her injuries. For that reason, we could not see into the back of the eye to operate, and we had to modify the procedure. We started by removing her damaged cornea and replacing it with a plastic, temporary cornea that allowed us to see the retina and operate. When we were done, we removed the plastic cornea and replaced it with a donor transplant cornea. Then we filled the back part of the eye with liquid silicone oil, replacing the natural jelly-like material called the vitreous gel. This helps to hold the retina in place, much like a cast contains a broken arm. The human retina is extremely fragile—a mere three human cells thick at its thickest point—and has the consistency of wet tissue paper. With the retina "splinted," we then leave it to heal until we remove the silicone oil three to six months later.

Ellen underwent three more procedures on her right eye, and one more on her left. We didn't hold out much hope for her left eye because she'd had quite a bit of damage to her optic nerve. The results for the right eye, however, were quite positive. A crew from *Nightline* came and filmed portions of the surgery and returned when she got her bandages off. Within three months of the procedure, Ellen could read 20/50 (when she stood twenty feet from an eye chart, she could see what a typical person would see at fifty feet), which is a pretty remarkable recovery.

Sadly, because of the damage that occurred in the time it took to reach that diagnosis, her retina deteriorated to the point where she lost the vision she had regained.

We're planning to operate on Ellen again as soon as we can fine-tune the procedures and technology required to deal with her injuries. Because we haven't ever actually done what Ellen's eyes require, however, I can't really offer any statistics or probability percentages of success.

Despite all the setbacks and months of waiting, Ellen Bomer is a remarkable person. She has a tremendously positive attitude about life and a positive spirit as well. When I first met her she had already accepted the fact that she was going to be blind for the rest of her life. And yet somehow she balanced that acceptance with hope that her vision would be restored. Then, after the surgery and restored vision, to have lost it again—I can't imagine how discouraging that must have been. Yet I never heard her complain, never heard her ask, "Why me?" For Ellen, life is so valuable; she's not going to waste a minute of it feeling sorry for herself. Not only that, she is without a doubt one of the most courageous people I've ever met. She's enriched my life in many ways and I'm proud to call her my friend.

Dr. Harold Snider, Ph.D.

In September of 1998, my ex-wife, Gail, was working at an agency for the blind in Washington, D.C., when Don Bomer came in looking for help for his wife, Ellen.

Gail called and told me Ellen had been blinded in the embassy attack in Nairobi. Because it had been an international incident, Gail thought the National Federation of the Blind (NFB) might want to get involved. Since I did quite a bit of consulting work for them at that time, I called them to discuss the possibility of helping her. Their response: "Of course, just do it."

Later, as my wife, Linda, and I rode over to Walter Reed Hospital to meet with Ellen, I said, "Linda, you need to know that if we can be of help to Ellen, this isn't a one-shot deal. We can't just walk in, give some advice, and walk away. I'll mentor her, work with her, and hang in there with her."

Linda agreed and understood what we were probably getting into as we proceeded to the hospital and made our way to Ellen's room.

It didn't take long for me to observe that Ellen's situation wasn't particularly good. At that point, for example, she couldn't put toothpaste on a toothbrush, and she couldn't use a cell phone. I made sure before I left that day, however, that she could do those things.

When we first talked, Ellen thought of blindness as an utter and complete tragedy; her notion of a blind person was someone who stood on a street corner with a cup and pencils. She was sure her life was basically over. Of course, not only was she blind, her ears and hands were damaged, as well. She told me she thought she had enough wood, metal, and glass in her to construct a building! All in all, she was feeling pretty sorry for herself.

The first thing we did, then, was to network her with other blind people, especially those who had experienced traumatic vision loss, individuals she could contact to answer questions and encourage her when she felt down.

As time went by, Linda and I and Don and Ellen really clicked. We have several things in common: All four of us had experienced divorce; we all had children who'd been a bit wayward; all of us were from the South; and all liked hot, spicy food. So, not only did I become Ellen's mentor, we all became fast friends.

By 1999, Ellen was attending the Louisiana Center for the Blind. Also that year, she and Don attended the NFB national convention—along with about three thousand other blind people. While we were there, I taught her how to travel on an escalator. She had told me she couldn't, because she was too frightened.

"Ellen," I said, "there's nothing to be afraid of if you do it right." I showed her how to approach and get off, and when we were done, she said, "Hey! There's nothing to this!"

Also at this time, my son, David, was filming Ellen for her appearance on *Nightline*. When I spoke with Ted Koppel, I told him that when I'd first met Ellen, she was below zero—not even on the scale—as far as being able to function. By the time of the broadcast, she was probably at about 50 percent. Now, however, she's capable of doing whatever needs to be done—from cooking to raising her granddaughter, to winning arguments with Don. She lives as a typical person who happens to have the disability of blindness.

In 2000–2001 Ellen granted me the rehabilitation contract with the Office of Workers' Compensation Program (OWCP) within the Department of Labor so she could get the equipment she needed to maintain her independence—a computer, a Braille printer, a Braille note-taker, and a variety of other aids and devices that the government could purchase. In that capacity, I handled the paperwork required to procure these items.

Don and Ellen are such decent people—you'll not hear them complain—and our country is so lucky to have people like them who serve.

Ellen has taken charge of her own destiny. She's made choices about employment, about where she lives, and about how she functions. She's doing a tremendous job of raising her granddaughter and running her household. Most of all, I've seen Ellen's faith carry her through the tough times she's faced.

Ellen came back from her injuries in a most extraordinary way. I hesitate to use words such as *bravery* and *courage*, but if there's anybody who's got guts and courage, it's Ellen and Don Bomer.

Last year we received a call informing us that Dr. Harold Snider passed away. He was my mentor in the ways of blindness, and our very dear and special friend. Harold was like a life preserver thrown to us as we floundered in an ocean of self-pity and doubt. He fought the good fight as my advocate for healthcare, stabilizing my life. His passing is a great loss to us personally as well as the global blind community. He was a mentor and friend to many around the world. May Jehovah bless and keep him until we meet again.

Mr. Art Kauffman

After church one Sunday almost three years ago, my wife Jan saw a gruff-looking big bear of a man sitting by himself at a table in the room where everyone gathers for coffee. She walked over and introduced herself to him. The man turned out to be Don Bomer. We did not meet Ellen on that occasion, but because Jan, Don, and I have all served in the military, we found common ground, really hitting it off together.

Our friendship cemented when Ellen and I joined what our church calls "Community of Hope," a program for laypeople to learn how to minister to those who are sick or grieving. Jan had talked to Ellen about participating, but Ellen wasn't sure how she would get to and from the training sessions and how she would complete the required reading.

When Jan relayed this to me, I said, "I'm willing to do whatever I can to help her if she really wants to make this happen." So I called Ellen and made the necessary arrangements.

Part of the training included prayer and daily Bible reading, which Ellen and I did together on the phone. (Due to circumstances, Jan dropped out of the training, but Ellen and I completed it.)

When the class ended, Ellen and I decided to continue our devotional times. For the past two years, we've connected by phone about five times a week for prayer and Scripture reading. We've actually read through the entire New Testament and a large portion of the Old. Recently, we've incorporated a book called *Nelson's New Illustrated Bible Manners and Customs* by Howard Vos, which gives insight—based on the Bible and the archaeological record—into government, religion, diet, family life, and so forth at each stage of biblical history. Along with that, we also read from the Rule of Benedict (a set of rules for monastics, written by Saint Benedict around 530 A.D.), which Ellen agreed to do as part of her training in Community of Hope.

Of course, I'm not sure how many people continue the required prayers and reading when the training's complete, but Ellen signed an agreement to do so, and she has every intention of following through with her commitment.

As I've gotten to know Ellen better, several things have impressed me. First, she's just so happy and positive. She said to me once, "When we bought this house, I hated the kitchen. It's so small—I had plans to rip it out and completely remodel it. But, you know, this kitchen is just the right size for a blind person." Being blind has changed her whole perspective on her life and circumstances. Also, Ellen's taking EFM, Education for Ministry, to expand and deepen her Bible knowledge. Her desire to learn and grow seems to be boundless. Then, for Don and Ellen to take on raising their granddaughter—these people are my heroes!

As far as the future, I'd love to see Ellen pursue public speaking, if she's so inclined. I've heard her speak, and she's got a God-given ability to communicate with passion, humor, and grace. I'm sure she could challenge and encourage many through her words.

I treasure Ellen's friendship. She has been and continues to be a blessing to my life.

Mrs. Eleanor Edwards

About three years ago, our church's Director of Christian Education approached me with a request. She said, "There's a person new to the church who needs a ride to Sunday school. She'd also like to bring her granddaughter who is living with her."

My husband and I were happy to make the drive, which is about twenty minutes from the church, so I called and made the arrangements, and that's how Ellen and I first got acquainted.

It didn't take long for my "transportation ministry" to blossom into a friendship, and now we get together every Thursday morning. We talk, of course, but I also read to her. My husband teaches our Sunday school class, so I read the study materials to Ellen so she can prepare for Sunday mornings. I also read various other books and magazines related to our shared interests. Sometimes we talk about the other church class we both attend, called Education for Ministry. Ellen has those materials on her computer, so her computer reads them aloud to her, but, of course, it doesn't actually discuss the concepts or pause to make sure she understands. However, Ellen has developed her memory to such an extent—the number of names, phone numbers, and so forth that she keeps in her head is astonishing—she is a quick learner and has little trouble with the class.

Both at church and at the Bomers' home, I've enjoyed watching Ellen with Allie. Allie's pretty strong-willed, especially when it comes to her wardrobe choices, but Ellen has a device that, when she swipes it across a shirt or dress, will tell her the color of the article of clothing. Once in a while, Allie will pull a fast one on Ellen. I remember one Sunday I said to Ellen, "I see Allie got to wear those boots to church after all, eh?"

Ellen replied, "She did?"

We laughed about it later, but I'm sure Allie got a stern reprimand on the way home from church that day!

Along with the device that's helped her arrange her clothing, Ellen's figured out several other ways of getting around her blindness. For example, when she wanted to go to the gym, she knew she would have to rely on her assistant for transportation there and back, as well as assistance with the various machines. To avoid all that hassle, for a while she used their long driveway as her "track," and simply did laps out to the road for her workout. It was relatively effective, but not very enjoyable!

Still, Ellen has said to me, "I just have to remember it takes me twice as long to do things." She's such an energetic go-getter, it's tough for her to have to take so much longer than a sighted person would to accomplish a task. Nevertheless, she's not bitter, and she's always experimenting, trying to find ways of improving her quality of life.

I really admire Ellen for her perseverance and her positive attitude, especially as she's waited month after month to undergo the next surgery that could restore her vision. Yet, she never loses hope, and I know she has complete trust in Dr. Witherspoon—and in God—that everything will happen at the right time. I'm sure God has a plan for her and I feel privileged to watch as it unfolds.

Ms. Tseghe Reade

I first met Ellen in Saudi Arabia in 1993. I left my home country of Eritrea on the east coast of Africa, due to the war there, and needed a job. Ellen needed a cook and housekeeper, so it was a good match. We got along quite well, and I worked for her until she went to Nairobi in 1998.

After the bombing and Ellen's early recovery in Washington, D.C., it was time for Don to go back to work, and they needed someone to assist her with her daily tasks. When they called, I was happy to come to the States to work with her again.

At first it was really hard. I cared for Ellen each day—which included picking glass out of her body. She cried almost every night for many weeks. I'm sure it must have been very scary to have been sighted one day and blind the next, with no warning. I also think it was so hard for her not to be able to do what she was used to doing, and to have to rely on someone for the smallest things. I did my best to reassure and encourage her, and most of the time she listened to me.

I stayed with her, then, until she went to the school for the blind in Louisiana.

One thing I admire about Ellen is her strength; she's a very strong person. She believes in God, and when she lost her sight, she came to accept it, and she worked through it. Then, when Allie came to live with her and Don, I was amazed at how well she handled taking care of a baby, even though she couldn't see.

Ellen is a wonderful example to all of us of a person who was faced with a horrible situation, walked through it, and became a better person in the end.

CHAPTER 14

" . . . BUT GOD MEANT IT FOR GOOD . . . "

WHEN JACOB DIED, Joseph's brothers were afraid that he would take revenge upon them. These are the words of Joseph to his brothers:

> Genesis 50:20: But as for you, you meant evil against me; *but* God meant it for good, in order to bring it about as it is this day, to save many people alive.[5]

So what good has come from the bombing? Grace, unmerited favor, is a gift from God that blesses me every day. I'm a different person today than before the bombing, and I would say I'm a better person.

When John was killed we filed suit against the trucking company, but I never sat down with the driver. The lawyers read me his deposition. He was only twenty-four years old and had a family. He never drove a commercial truck again and wouldn't even drive the truck away from the accident. At the time I just wanted someone to say that my son's life counted for something, but I never got that. I just felt sorry for the truck driver.

Because of my near-death experiences, many things have changed since the terrorist bombing. I was able to say goodbye to my son, John. I now know there was no place for him on earth, but he is safe with God.

People ask me how I can be so positive about life after my experiences at the hands of terrorists. I tell them that I *KNOW* God knows me by name. God has always been in my life, but not always at the forefront. How can I have any negatives in my life when God has given me life and knows me by name? I'm a better person because I'm not so materialistic. I don't respond to appearances because I'm blind, and I place much more emphasis on relationships. Besides, if you want people to help you, you can't act ugly.

I'm not afraid to die and truly know that my recovery from close encounters was for a purpose. Because of my ordeal and my personal relationship with the love and peace of God, Don became a believer and accepted Jesus Christ as his Savior. We are raising Allie; and Michael, Allie's father, has become the loving and caring son that I always prayed for. I was meant to do this. The terrorists meant it for evil, but God meant it for good.

RESOURCES

S EVERAL RESOURCES FOR the blind and visually impaired have been mentioned throughout this book. The following contact information was accurate at the time of publication.

Aids and Appliances for the Blind:

National Federation of the Blind Products:

- NFB Independence Market:
  http://www.nfb.org/nfb/Independence_Market.asp/
- Resource List for Aids and Appliances:
  http://www.nfb.org/nfb/ResourceList_
  AidsAndAppliances.asp

Kurzweil-National Federation of the Blind (KNFB) Reader: A combination cell phone and camera; takes a photo of any document and reads it back (Shipped with English and Spanish, other languages available).

http://www.knfbreader.com/

Library of Congress/National Library Service:

Provides books and periodicals on tape and readers to any American who is unable to read.
http://www.loc.gov/nls/

National Federation of the Blind (NFB):

1800 Johnson Street
Baltimore, MD 21230
Phone: 410-659-9314
Fax: 410-685-5653
http://www.nfb.org/nfb/Default.asp

NFB Affiliated Schools for the Blind:

Louisiana Center for the Blind
101 South Trenton Street
Ruston, LA 71270
Phone: 800-234-4166
http://www.lcb-ruston.com/

Colorado Center for the Blind
2233 West Shepperd Ave.
Littleton, CO 80120
Phone: 303-778-1130
Toll Free: 800-401-4632
FAX: 303-778-1598
http://www.cocenter.org/

Blind, Inc.
100 East 22nd St.
Minneapolis, MN 55404
Phone: 612-872-0100
Fax: 612-872-9358
http://www.blindinc.org/

NFB-NEWSLINE®:

866-504-7300

http://www.nfb.org/nfb/newspapers_by_phone.asp

NFB State and Local Organizations:

http://www.nfb.org/nfb/State_and_Local_Organizations.asp

Organ and Tissue Donation:

- http://en.wikipedia.org/wiki/Organ_donation
- http://www.mayoclinic.com/health/organ-donation/FL00077
- http://www.organdonor.gov/
- http://www.organtransplants.org/

My Website:

www.ellen-bomer.com

My Blog:

http://ellenbomer.authorweblog.com

ENDNOTES

1. Referenced: ABC *Nightline* press release, © 1999 by Disney.

2. Referenced: ABC *Nightline* Ellen Bomer transcripts, August 5 and 6, 1999 © 1999 Disney.

3. Trial transcript: USA v. Osama bin Laden et al, May 1, 2001 (pp. 5223–5230), http://cryptome.org/usa-v-ubl-37.htm.

4. Referenced: Associated Press article by Pat Milton, "Blinded American Waits for Justice," May 4, 2001, © 2001 Associated Press.

5. Photograph taken at the Nairobi, Kenya, United States Embassy © 1999 by Danny DeVito. Used by permission.

6. Photographs taken at Louisiana Center for the Blind and at the National Federation of the Blind Convention © 1999 by David Snider. Used by permission.

7. Photographs taken at the Nairobi, Kenya, United States Embassy © 1999 by Worley Lee Reed. Used by permission.

8. Excerpt from photograph of the St. Stephen's Episcopal Church Junior Choir © 2008 by Maria Mullins. Used by permission.

9. "Who Did This?" poem by Bessie M. Campbell © 1999. Used by permission.

All information included follows Fair Use sect. 107 of 2009 Copyright Act.

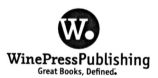

CPSIA information can be obtained at www.ICGtesting.com

224415LV00001B/3/P

9 781414 113661